BACH FLOWER
REMEDIES
f   BEGINNERS

A Comprehensive Guide to the Bach Flower Remedies

Every day we are subjected to thousands of distractions, stressors, and pollutants. These myriad influences can wear down our natural defenses and cause frustration, tension, and even physical illness. The thirty-eight Bach Flower Remedies are a safe and natural solution to the challenges of life in the twenty-first century. The remedies purify and balance the internal energy system, which in turn heals existing health problems—and can even help prevent future problems from manifesting!

At the end of the day, are you often left feeling overwhelmed by too much pressure and responsibility? The Elm remedy encourages clear thinking and boosts inner strength. Are you trapped in a cycle of repetitive or destructive behavior? Chestnut Bud will help you learn from your experiences and control negative or repetitive behavior. Have you suffered an extreme shock or trauma, such as surgery or a serious illness? The combination Rescue Remedy will soothe your mind and emotions while stimulating physical regeneration.

Bach Flower Remedies for Beginners is a comprehensive guide to the use of these powerful healing tools. Whether you're new to alternative healing or an experienced practitioner, this book is a valuable healing resource.

About the Author

David F. Vennells, a qualified reflexologist and Reiki teacher, has used the Bach Flower Remedies for almost ten years as a complement to his work with Reiki and reflexology, creating a complete system of healing for the body and mind He discovered the effectiveness of the remedies while suffering from chronic fatigue syndrome. He currently resides and practices in northwest England.

To Write to the Author

If you wish to contact the author or would like more information about this book, please write to the author in care of Llewellyn Worldwide, and we will forward your request. Both the author and publisher appreciate hearing from you. Llewellyn Worldwide cannot guarantee that every letter written to the author can be answered, but all will be forwarded. Please write to:

David F. Vennells
℅ Llewellyn Worldwide
P.O. Box 64383, 0-7387-0047-9
St. Paul, MN 55164-0383, U.S.A.

Please enclose a self-addressed, stamped envelope for reply, or $1.00 to cover costs. If outside the U.S.A., enclose international postal reply coupon.

Many of Llewellyn's authors have websites with additional information and resources. For more information, please visit our website at
http://www.llewellyn.com

BACH FLOWER REMEDIES
for BEGINNERS

38 Essences that Heal
from Deep Within

David F. Vennells

2001
Llewellyn Publications
St. Paul, Minnesota 55164-0383

FIRST EDITION
First printing, 2001

Cover design: Zulma Davila
Dr. Edward Bach photo: Courtesy of The Bach Centre, Sotwell, England. The
    photograph of Dr. Edward Bach is a registered trademark of Bach Flower
    Remedies Ltd., Oxfordshire, England.
Editing and book design: Christine Snow
Illustration, pg. 85: Kevin Brown
Medicine Buddha illustration: Courtesy of Tharpa Publications © 1990.
    Illustrated by Andy Weber

Library of Congress Cataloging-in-Publication Data
Vennells, David F.
    Bach flower remedies for beginners: 38 essences that heal from
        deep within / David F. Vennells.
            p. cm.
    Includes bibliographical references and index.
    ISBN 0-7387-0047-9
    1. Flowers–Therapeutic use. 2. Homeopathy–Materia medica
        and therapeutics. I. Title.
    RX615.F55 V46 2001
    615'.321–dc21   00-048388

Llewellyn Publications
A Division of Llewellyn Worldwide, Ltd.
P.O. Box 64383, Dept. 0-7387-0047-9
St. Paul, MN 55164-0383
www.llewellyn.com

Printed in the United States of America

Other Books by David F. Vennells

Reiki for Beginners
(Llewellyn Publications, 1999)

Upcoming Books

Reflexology for Beginners
(Llewellyn Publications, 2001)

Acknowledgments

Many thanks to everyone who has contributed
to the making of this book—especially to Dr. Edward
Bach, for his gift of healing remedies and for his great
example of kindness and compassion for others.

Special thanks always to Mum and Dad.

Also to Judy Howard at the Dr. Edward Bach
Centre and everyone who helps the Centre
in its wonderful healing work.

Thanks also to Nancy Mostad and
Christine Snow at Llewellyn Publications
for their support and encouragement, which
helps make writing a real pleasure.

Deepest thanks for the constant care, patience,
and kindness of my spiritual guide and teachers.

Contents

Note

The practices and techniques described in this book should not be used as an alternative to professional medical treatment. This book does not attempt to give any medical diagnosis, treatment, prescription, or suggestion for medication in relation to any human disease, pain, injury, deformity, or physical or mental condition.

The author and publisher of this book are not responsible in any manner whatsoever for any injury which may occur through following the instructions contained herein. It is recommended that before beginning any remedy treatment, you consult your physician to determine whether you are medically, physically, and mentally fit to undertake this course of practice.

Introduction

The Bach Flower Remedies are a profoundly powerful force for good and yet so simple and accessible that anyone can use them effectively with only a little study and a good heart. Dr. Edward Bach discovered these wonderful healing remedies. He wanted nothing more than to help others in whatever way he could. This pure, altruistic motivation was the key to his success in discovering and developing the Bach Flower Remedies. If we can understand and develop a little of this pure motivation within us it will form the perfect basis on which to practice this special form of healing therapy.

Once you have some knowledge of the remedies and how to use them, I encourage you to begin taking them right away without extensive study. The quickest way to learn is through experience. Look through the quick reference guide to each remedy in chapter 8, and make a list of the remedies that you think might be appropriate for yourself or someone you would like to treat. Then read the in-depth description of each of those remedies before making your final decision. Once you are comfortable with your selections, buy the remedies and use them. This is a good way of becoming familiar with the remedies and to slowly build up a collection of them, if you do not want to buy them all at once.

Many people would say that we are living in an age of superficiality, materialism, pollution, and spiritual poverty. I am not sure how Dr. Bach would react to the world today. I think he would be deeply sad but, perhaps, not surprised to see so much unhappiness and discontentment, often in the midst of so much wealth. Dr. Bach stressed the importance of inner healing—healing the whole person, not just the physical aspect. He understood human nature and he knew that healing the body without healing the mind was pointless. Quite simply, if we are not healthy and happy on the inside, we will have a poor quality of life even if we have good physical health and good external conditions. His message to us was to develop and nurture our inner nature and to find happiness from a continuous and lasting source. He developed the remedies primarily to help us achieve these goals as well as physical healing.

I hope the essence of this book communicates some of the doctor's special views on life. As a practicing Buddhist, I have noticed many similarities between Dr. Bach's philosophy and the teachings of Buddha. There is so much common ground, so much wisdom and compassion in both, I felt sure that other people interested in the Bach remedies would benefit greatly from looking at the remedies from a Buddhist perspective.

This is in no way designed to challenge anyone's beliefs or faith in other religions; we definitely do not need to be Buddhist to benefit from Buddha's teachings. I only hope this wisdom will enrich and deepen your understanding and experience of your own faith or spiritual path to personal growth and help you to gain clearer insight into Dr. Bach's work.

Although this book is designed as a beginner's guide, I think there is also a great deal of information that experienced Bach flower practitioners will find fascinating and invaluable.

Dr. Bach felt that he was building on the work of his predecessors, such as Samuel Hahnemann, the founder of homeopathy. In an address to a medical society given in 1931, Dr. Bach said:

> *Do not think for one moment that one is detracting from Hahnemann's work, on the contrary, he pointed out the great fundamental laws, the basis; but he had only one life, and had he continued his work longer no doubt he would have progressed along these lines. We are merely advancing his work, and carrying it to the next natural stage.*

If Dr. Bach felt that he was building on the work of Samuel Hahnemann and had no hesitation in saying that, then what is the next natural stage that leads on from where Dr. Bach left off? If Dr. Bach were alive today, into what areas of health and healing would he be researching? How can we build on what Dr. Bach achieved? He felt that his healing system was complete and that it did not need alterations or additions. The results of many years' experience have shown this to be true. It is doubtful that humankind will ever find cures more natural, gentle, and effective.

There are, however, areas in the philosophy of healing relating to the Bach system that could be clarified, and I feel it would be these areas that Dr. Bach would be channeling his energies and publishing his findings. For example, what the real cause of disease is, the true nature or essence of the remedies, how the Bach remedies actually work to cure illness, how we can practically use the remedies to prevent illness, understanding the nature of the mind in relation to the remedies, and using this wisdom to find inner peace and, eventually, freedom from all kinds of suffering. These areas and many others are covered in this book, and I hope that these subjects inspire beginners and experienced practitioners to see the Bach system of healing in a new and clearer light.

I have personally gained great benefit from the remedies, and I have seen the lives of many people healed and transformed by using them. Reading and writing about the life and work of Dr. Bach has been a great inspiration and learning experience for me. I hope that some of the faith and enthusiasm I have in the remedies is passed on to readers so that many more people will be encouraged to use the remedies and that the great work of Dr. Bach is passed on and continued for many generations to come.

I wish you good health and great happiness.

One

The Life of Edward Bach

Edward Bach was born September 24, 1886, in Moseley, a village near Birmingham, England. He was the eldest son of three children and by all accounts, apart from suffering from poor health in the first few years of his life, he led a fairly normal childhood.

He was a friendly child with an intelligent sense of humor and a great interest in people and everything around him. He had a special love of all things "natural" and seemed happiest and most content when outdoors, playing in the fields, woods, ponds, and streams around his home village or while on vacation with his family in the Welsh countryside.

1

Dr. Bach was sensitive, intuitive, and sometimes intense as a child. He had an unusually high level of concentration and loved reading about and studying the natural world. He often went through periods of quiet contemplation and, like most children, he asked questions about life, the universe—everything. Why are we here? What is our purpose? Where do we go when we die? Why do people get ill?

Wales was a special place to him, a hidden gem. He returned there many times throughout his life. While in Wales as a young man, he often went for long walks through the villages, fields, and over the mountains, enjoying the natural surroundings and studying the flora and fauna native to that country.

Wales has a long history, a unique culture, and many holy places with connections to the Celtic and Druid religions and the early Christian saints and mystics. The young Edward must have been fascinated by the stories surrounding these people and places and the well-known myths and legends of dragons, knights, wizards, holy beings, and healers of Welsh tradition.

The Bach Flower Remedies are often thought of as English in origin, but they are as much a product of Wales. The first three remedies were found in Wales and Dr. Bach did much of his thinking, researching, and writing in Wales. This country had a special place in his heart; its effect on his childhood and its sustaining influence throughout his life made great contributions to the culmination of his life's work.

As a boy, Dr. Bach dreamed of finding a universal cure for all illnesses, and that one day he would be able to heal people just as Jesus had done—simply by touch. He had great compassion for animals and humans alike. Many children have similar fantasies, and these altruistic notions are often dulled by the process of having to conform to the rules of a cynical society that discourages such flights of fancy. Dr. Bach never lost his innocence and idealism despite his intelligence and superb analytical mind. He was always open to the possibilities of the

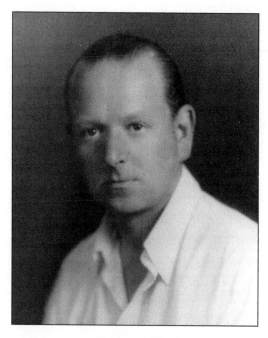

Dr. Edward Bach

unknown, and he was always interested in the esoteric and spiritual aspects of human beings.

This need to help others grew throughout his childhood and became so strong that he knew, even from an early age, that he would become a doctor. Ultimately his compassion for others was the great power that fueled his search for a gentle, effective, yet powerful method for healing the mind and body. There is no doubt that his dedication to this aim and the eventual success of his endeavors was due to this simple wish to lose himself in the service of others. Perhaps it seemed to him that the culmination of his spiritual path or purpose in life was to give his life in this way. Some say that the greatest or purest happiness and contentment comes from living in such a selfless way. Certainly many spiritual traditions advocate this way of life, and most of the holy men and women of the world's religions have these qualities.

There were many instances during his career when he felt an overwhelming sense of compassion for his patient. He would touch them and instantly feel a flow of healing energy from "above" and within himself to the patient. The patient gained great benefit and relief from this "treatment" and often was completely cured of his or her illness. There is an obvious similarity here with the healings of Jesus, Buddha, and many other great healers. They lived their lives to benefit others, and they were always motivated by great compassion.

Dr. Bach left school at sixteen and worked for his father for a few years in his brass foundry business. He tried his hand at the various jobs available within the business, from heavy manual work to office duties. He also worked as a traveling salesman for a while, but his honesty and constant wish to help others as much as he could did not make him a very successful salesman, although he was very popular with his customers. Perhaps these years gave him valuable insight into human nature. He must have rubbed shoulders with many different types of people from all walks of life.

He greatly yearned for the natural surroundings of his beloved countryside instead of being holed up in a stuffy office or in the heat and grime of the foundry. Although he must have felt like a square peg in a round hole later in life, he may have looked back on these times and realized their value in helping him determine what was and what was not his right path in life.

His interest in the medical profession grew, and after a short time of considering a life in the church, he set his heart on becoming a doctor. Again, it was his overwhelming desire to aid the sick that helped him decide. He still desired to heal in the same simple and effective ways of Jesus and other religious healers, but he also felt that he should investigate all methods of healing, including conventional medicine, so he would have more tools and knowledge with which to help others. Then he could discard what did not work or what seemed to do more harm than good.

Supported by his parents, Dr. Bach began his medical studies at Birmingham University College Hospital, where he graduated in 1912. A year later he earned two additional medical degrees, and in 1914 he also received a diploma of public health at Cambridge.

His years of study were difficult. He disliked being dependent on his parents, so he worked various part-time jobs to supplement his income. He continued to study spiritual matters and other forms of healing like herbalism, which he felt were overlooked by the medical profession. He also began to realize that conventional medicine was, in fact, primitive in many ways and often impotent in the face of chronic illness. He came into contact with much suffering during his medical training that must have caused him to question the validity of many of the medical practices he was learning. But he did successfully finish his formal training and became a fully qualified medical doctor. Perhaps if he hadn't, the Bach remedies today would not have such a good reputation or be so widely used.

Throughout his medical training he began to formulate some vague notions regarding the real causes and cures of disease, as he felt sure that modern medicine was missing the point. He had not forgotten his childhood dreams of discovering special medicines that would cure any illness and restore peace of mind and good health. He certainly learned a lot about the way different people react to illness and the qualities that make some patients more likely to make a full and swift recovery.

It became obvious to him from early on that there was a strong link between the healing process and the state of mind of the patient. It was not long before he began to think that mental attitude might have a more direct, even causative role, in the early stages of illness. In fact, by the end of his medical training, Dr. Bach felt that if he was going to successfully continue his research into the real causes of disease he would have to "un-learn" much of what he had been taught at medical school.

His first job was as an emergency room doctor, although he had to give this up after a few months due to poor health, probably from overwork. After a swift recovery, he began a general practice in London that quickly became busy. His interest in searching for the real causes of illness led him to study immunology as an assistant bacteriologist at University College Hospital while still running his general practice.

His health was generally poor, and he was refused entry into the armed forces during World War I. However, he was able to help thousands of war casualties that came through his hospital. Toward the end of the war, he became very ill due to overwork and suffered a severe hemorrhage that nearly killed him. Many of his colleagues were quite surprised to see him make a full recovery and return to work. He felt that what really carried him through his illness was the belief that he had a definite purpose to fulfill in life. At that time he was making progress covering new ground, and he thought these advances might lead to something really special, although he had no clear idea what that might be.

In 1919, Dr. Bach was appointed pathologist and bacteriologist at the London Homeopathic Hospital, where he stayed until 1922. He continued his work in bacteriology and combined his findings with his new knowledge of homeopathy to produce the Seven Bach Nosodes, successful bacteria-based cures for different types of chronic illness, which are still in use today. Before he came to the London Homeopathic Hospital, he had established seven groups of intestinal bacteria that were prevalent in patients with certain chronic illnesses. He was able to formulate successful cures for these, and his results improved greatly having mastered the methods of preparing homeopathic remedies.

Before becoming interested in homeopathy, Dr. Bach had already noted that patients with the same illness responded better to different remedies. He noticed that people with similar personalities responded well to the same remedies even when their illnesses were totally different. In fact, he could often prescribe the right remedy simply by observing a patient's temperament and disposition without physically examining the patient. To find a system of medicine that had this principal of diagnosis at its heart was a truly wonderful discovery for Dr. Bach.

Dr. Bach must have been greatly impressed by the works of Samuel Hahnemann, the founder of homeopathy. There are obvious similarities between them. Their motives were both strong and true, and they were not afraid to stand alone in their beliefs that the natural world had a lot to offer the medical field. They were both ahead of their time as great thinkers and philosophers. They also had a strong belief in the innate spiritual qualities of humans and that therein lie the simple key to health and happiness for all.

In Dr. Bach's book *Heal Thyself* he says:

One of the exceptions to the materialistic methods in modern [medical] science is that of the great Hahnemann, the founder of Homeopathy, who with his realization of the beneficent love of the Creator and of the Divinity which resides within man, by studying the mental attitude of his patients towards life, environment and their respective diseases, sought to find in the herbs of the field and in the realms of nature the remedy which would not only heal their body but at the same time would uplift their mental outlook. May his science be extended and developed by those true physicians who have the love of humanity at heart.

Throughout his career he was aware that his intuition or inner wisdom was a very powerful and useful tool. He often employed such skills to guide and sustain his research, especially at times when he was breaking new ground or looking for a new line of reasoning. He was a very spiritual man, although not necessarily religious. His trust and faith in this natural relationship with God, his own intuitive wisdom or "higher nature" increasingly became the guiding force in his life and work. As this aspect of his nature became more prominent, he felt an increasing urgency to set his sights on his lifelong ambition to discover and perfect cures that were far more effective and advanced than any others currently available.

By this time he strongly felt that conventional medicine was not going in the right direction; that the causes of disease were seen mainly as a physical problem and in no way related to a patient's personality or mental state.

It seemed to him that homeopathy was addressing this issue very effectively through its system of diagnosis, which directly related to the patient as a whole person or organism, not just a body. In *Heal Thyself* he says:

> *Disease will never be cured or eradicated by present materialistic methods, for the simple reason that disease in its origin is not material.*

In fact, Dr. Bach goes on to say:

> *The modern trend of medical science, by misinterpreting the true nature of the disease and concentrating it in materialistic terms in the physical body, has enormously increased its power, firstly, by distracting the thoughts of people from its true origin and hence form the effective method of attack, and secondly, by localizing it in the body, thus obscuring true hope of recovery and raising a mighty disease complex of fear, which never should have existed.*

He saw that new illnesses were always arising and derivations of existing illnesses were making some medicines useless. He knew that this would always be the case unless medicine could penetrate the heart of the matter.

After using the Seven Bach Nosodes for several years, he was able to clearly identify seven personality types that responded the most effectively to this type of treatment. It was a quick and effective way of prescribing and saved a lot of time and trouble for both the doctor and patient. He wrote papers and gave lectures about his discoveries and many people began to recognize him as a leader in homeopathic and conventional medicine. He was always open about his research and discoveries and keen for as many people to benefit from whatever work he had done. He continued his general practice during this time and often refused payment for his services when people couldn't afford it. The money he did earn went to further his research or support his staff.

While continuing to clarify the personality types that responded well to the nosodes, he also began to notice other personality types. He also felt that the remedies for the nosode types might be more effective if they came from a more natural source rather than from a homeopathic potency of the original diseased material. This is where his great love of nature and knowledge of wildflowers and trees came in.

The point at which Dr. Bach began to look for natural remedies to replace the Seven Bach Nosodes marked a powerful turning point in his life. It was as if he was taking the first steps outside the boundaries of conventional and homeopathic medicine. Although he processed or "potentized" the first remedies homeopathically, he was not specifically looking for homeopathic remedies to replace the nosodes. He was open to whatever he might find, whatever they might be, and wherever he might find them.

Two

Discovering the New Medicine

In 1928, Dr. Bach began to search for new natural remedies to replace the seven nosodes. When he first began to potentize plant remedies, he discovered that they were of a positive polarity whereas the nosodes were of a negative polarity. It was this negative polarity that made them so effective. Following on from this, he thought that if he would be able to find a new method for capturing the special healing qualities of these plants in a remedy with reversed polarity, he would have found a truly potent system of natural medicine. At that time he had no idea what form this new method of potentization might take, although he knew it would have to be pure and natural with as little man-made interference as possible. If a simple but effective system of herbal cures could be found covering the whole range of illnesses, using simple personality-based diagnosis, then this system could be easily practiced by anyone.

He also felt that healing should not be the sole prerogative of the medical profession. Patients should take a more active and responsible role.

The natural world is full of countless plants with healing qualities and many have healing potential yet to be discovered. Dr. Bach spent all his spare time studying existing natural remedies and making countless field trips to the countryside to study these plants in their natural surroundings. These excursions also gave his mind the openness and peace it required to develop the inner clarity needed to "see" and "feel" the special healing qualities of each plant. However, he could not find suitable remedies that worked as well as the nosodes, yet still he was convinced he was on the right track.

During this time, he also began to clarify the personality groups for which certain remedies might be particularly helpful. He spent much time studying human nature—his patients, friends, and colleagues, even people he met in the street or in the park. He watched their mannerisms, the way they spoke, the way they reacted to certain situations such as illness and good or bad news. He studied how they dealt with everyday situations and what their general outlook on life was and how this affected their quality of life. He began to see there were more personality types or groups than he had previously thought, and that most people fell within one of these groups.

Although he was not yet on the way to discovering appropriate remedies for all of these personality types, he felt that if he could identify these additional groups successfully, then the process of diagnosis would be much simpler and effective. He also noticed that people with similar personality types reacted in a similar way when ill; some would become depressed, some would become impatient, some would strive to get well, some would ignore their symptoms, while others would pretend to be coping well.

In the early autumn of 1929, he felt a strong intuitive urge to go to Wales on a search for new remedies. It was not long before he found two particular specimens that seemed to carry some special healing qualities: Impatiens and Mimulus. He found them growing in profusion by a mountain stream, high up where the air was pure and where there was an abundance of vibrant life force energy in the rocks and water. He prepared them both as herbal and homeopathic remedies to be used in place of two of the nosode remedies. He prescribed them according to the patient's temperament: Mimulus for those who were principally frightened or very nervous, and Impatiens for those who were easily irritated or impatient. The results were excellent. He was both pleased and excited that his hard work was beginning to show concrete results. Later that year he began to use Clematis to replace another one of the nosodes. This remedy produced good results in patients who were of a generally dreamy and light-headed disposition.

Perhaps these positive results energized Dr. Bach and confirmed his feelings that nature could provide all the remedies needed to restore good health naturally, safely, and easily. He must have felt as if he was on the verge of something very special.

As soon as he was convinced of the value of the three new remedies, he published a paper outlining their good qualities and how they might be used, so that others could benefit from them as soon as possible.

Toward the end of 1929, Dr. Bach reached a crossroads in his life. He knew that if he was going to succeed in his wish to bring about new attitudes and methods to healing the sick, he would have to completely discard anything that was holding him back. Many of his colleagues were interested in his ideas, but many also thought that he was moving too far away from conventional medicine. They thought that his considerable intelligence and medical knowledge would be far better served if he were to concentrate more on advancing his career in conventional medicine. However, he knew that if he did not have the courage and faith to follow his heart, then all that he had dreamed of since childhood would be lost. Now was not the time for faint hearts. He decided to leave London in 1930 and devote all his time to researching the flower remedies.

Perhaps in his heart he also knew that time was running out. Maybe he sensed that if he did not act now then there would not be a second chance. As it happened, from the time he began this "new life" he would only have six more years to live. In that time he would have to do the work of several lifetimes in order to accomplish his dream.

After leaving London he headed for his beloved Wales. It was probably a great relief for him to leave the city and, perhaps, symbolic of the beginnings of his inner journey that would reveal great truths and healing revelations. He walked many miles, day after day, week after week, always looking for suitable plants to add to his list of healers, plants that were of a special "higher order" and that stood out from the others as having special qualities. He became very sensitive to the subtle vibrations and internal life force energies of plants. No doubt this sensitivity also greatly assisted his understanding of the human condition and in the discovery of more personality groups for which he looked for appropriate remedies.

During his travels, he was also looking within himself for the divine guidance and inspiration that would manifest itself as inner spiritual revelations and outer discoveries of the remedies. He was traveling toward God and the outer manifestation of this spiritual path was the remedies used today. As well as possessing their own innate healing qualities, these remedies must also be blessed by Dr. Bach's own love and compassion toward others, a direct emanation of his compassionate soul.

Dr. Bach looked at many different plants and examined them in detail both analytically and intuitively. He studied their size, shape, color, taste, smell, favorite soil types, and other conditions that caused them to thrive or struggle. He eliminated many from his search simply by using his highly developed senses, even those which had traditionally been used as healing remedies. Just by holding the flower in his hand or placing it on his tongue, he could directly experience the good or bad effects it caused on the body and mind. He began to understand that it was the actual flower of the plant that held the highest vibrational healing quality, and that this energy seemed most potent at the time of year when the blooms were most profuse. He did not yet know how to capture this healing essence of the flower in the form of a usable remedy.

The First Flower Remedies

One morning in the late spring of 1930, while walking through a field heavy with dew, it occurred to him that the dew contained within the head of the flower might somehow receive and hold the special healing qualities of the flower. He also thought that the dew might be even more powerful if "energized" by direct sunlight while still on the flower. Excited by this revelation, he placed some dew directly on his tongue. The effects were immediate and powerful. He felt blessed and uplifted both mentally and physically. Suddenly all he had been working toward became clear, and he knew that he had discovered something truly remarkable.

He also discovered that dew that had not been in direct sunlight was not very potent, so he deduced that the action of the sun was a major factor in "drawing out" the high vibrational healing life force energy of the plant.

Dr. Bach realized that it was the combination of the flower, water, fresh air, and direct sunlight that created the best results. This "dew" remedy would be a manifestation of the four elements in their purest form: fire as the sunlight, the clean country air, water as the dew, and earth as the healing plant. Nothing could be simpler, purer, or more potent than the combination of these special qualities.

The next task for him was to find a way to duplicate this natural process that would allow him to collect large quantities of the potentized water. Obviously he would never be able to collect enough dew to fulfill this task, and the dew evaporated quickly in direct sunlight.

He collected enough of one type of flower and floated them in a glass bowl of pure water collected from a mountain stream. He then left it in the morning sun for two to three hours. His thought was that the water would absorb the healing qualities of the flowers just as the dew had done. To his delight, this "sun method" worked perfectly to harness the healing potential of the plant, and the first nineteen Bach Flower Remedies were all prepared in this way. He was convinced that the power of this method lay in its simplicity and purity.

He stayed in Wales to continue to perfect his sun method and also wrote his now-famous first book, *Heal Thyself.* In mid-1930, he moved to Cromer, a small town on the north coast of Norfolk, where he stayed until the spring of 1931. Over the next two years, he discovered the rest of the plants that would become known as the Twelve Healers and prepared them using the sun method. He found them in Wales, around Cromer and the Norfolk area, and also some in the Thames Valley, Sussex, and Kent.

He loved Cromer very much and would return there every winter when it was no longer possible to find new plants elsewhere because of the season. He used the winters to continue his research into the personality group theory and to practice his new method of healing on the local people. While he did spend some time in London, he found that he could not stay in the city for long periods. His highly sensitized state caused him to become physically ill and mentally stressed by the urban surroundings. Once he was back in Cromer or in the countryside, his health would return quickly.

He found Cromer to be an excellent place to advance his group personality theory as there were many types of people there; some were on holiday relaxing, some working for the holiday season, as well as local fishermen and farmers, and lots of children and adults and families. Many of them came to him when it became known that he was a doctor, and it was not long before his successful plant remedies became well known and appreciated.

The Twelve Healers

The Twelve Healers were prescribed for people with the following dispositions:

1.	Fear	Mimulus
2.	Terror	Rock Rose
3.	Mental torture/worry	Agrimony
4.	Indecision	Scleranthus
5.	Indifference/boredom	Clematis
6.	Doubt/discouragement	Gentian
7.	Overconcern	Chicory
8.	Weakness	Centaury
9.	Self-distrust	Cerato
10.	Impatience	Impatiens
11.	Overenthusiasm	Vervain
12.	Pride/aloofness	Water Violet

When he was convinced of the value of the Twelve Healers, he freely shared his discoveries with whomever was interested. He published papers and gave lectures on this new medicine whenever possible and continued using the remedies with great success.

Of the Twelve Healers, the only one not native to England or Wales was Cerato. This plant originated from Tibet, "the land of the snows." It is prescribed for those who suffer from self-doubt, those who need to trust and develop their own inner wisdom. (It is interesting to note that Tibet is synonymous with the Wisdom of the Buddhas.)

The Four Helpers

Although Dr. Bach was quite happy with his discoveries, he continued to find more personality types that he felt were not sufficiently represented by the Twelve Healers. In January 1933, he began to think about the possibility of a new series of remedies. These would be for those states of mind that were persistently negative and for those patients who felt helpless. This next group of remedies were called the Four Helpers:

13.	Gorse	Extreme hopelessness
14.	Oak	Those who never give up
15.	Heather	Self-obsessed
16.	Rock Water	Too strict and hard on self

He found the appropriate type of Heather in Wales, close to the spot where he found the first three remedies. Rock Water, the only nonplant remedy, was simply collected from a holy well renowned for its healing qualities in a previous age. This remedy can be made using any *pure* water source that has a special atmosphere or sense of peace surrounding it.

Having found these four remedies, he still felt that the collection was still incomplete, so he went on to find more:

17.	Wild Oat	Those looking for direction/purpose
18.	Olive	Physical and mental exhaustion
19.	Vine	Very strong, dominating, leaders

The Vine and Olive remedies were prepared for him by friends living in Switzerland and Italy. Perhaps Dr. Bach thought that if they were potentized in a country where they grew naturally, then this would be beneficial to the remedy. The Wild Oat remedy was found shortly after Dr. Bach took permanent residence at a small rented house called Mount Vernon in Sotwell, a small village near Wallingford in Berkshire. This place is still known as the Bach Flower Centre today and is the center of worldwide activities of the Bach Flower Foundation. This small, humble residence became very special to Dr. Bach, and he spent more time there than anywhere else until he died. He became well known and loved in the village. Many people who are interested in the Bach remedies or who want to develop a closer connection with Dr. Bach visit Mount Vernon. It is still a special place thanks to the care and commitment of those who are carrying on the doctor's work there.

In his first few weeks there, he wrote a short book called *The Twelve Healers and Seven Helpers*. After a short time he became very busy with patients. He had also begun releasing the remedies for use by other doctors, homeopaths, herbalists, and the general public, and he received many new inquiries and letters telling of excellent results.

His own healing abilities were often used, sometimes restoring good health by simply touching a patient or placing his hands on the problem area. Although he never knew when this would happen, he was always quick to play down his role, always attributing any such action to God's kindness. His powers of intuition and clairvoyance also became more acute, and it would be

these special qualities that would prove to be vital in discovering the next nineteen remedies.

A few days before finding each remedy, he would suffer from the negative state of mind that the remedy
cured. Sometimes they were very severe and the immense
suffering he endured during that time was eased only by
the presence and constant care of his good friend Nora
Weeks. Sometimes the state of mind would be accompanied by physical symptoms, at times even having problems walking a short distance.

The first of the remaining nineteen remedies he
found was Cherry Plum, used for those who fear they
are on the brink of insanity or a mental breakdown, a
fear of losing control. For a few days before finding this
remedy, this was how Dr. Bach felt. When he found the
Cherry Plum remedy it was early spring 1935, and the
tree was not yet in full bloom. He had to find another
way of tapping into its healing potential. He did this by
collecting a number of smaller branches with buds and
flowers on them and boiling these in a large pan of
water for one hour. He strained the remaining liquid
and placed a few drops on his tongue. The relief from
his agonizing symptoms was immediate, and by the next
day he was fully recovered.

Most of the remaining remedies were found and prepared in the same way. He was able to complete the system of remedies in August 1935. Because of his extensive
knowledge of the plant world and his great sensitivity, he
was able to identify the new remedies quickly, usually
within a few days of developing the symptoms. These

severe symptoms were the guides he needed to help him see which personality groups he had yet to discover or for which he did not have a remedy. Despite this constant strain, hard work, and illness, he never gave up or lost heart. He knew he was on to something special and that if he gave his all, many people would benefit from his discoveries. That was his main thought and motivation for continuing his work.

When the last of the thirty-eight remedies had been found, he stopped developing serious mental and physical symptoms, and he knew his work was complete. This must have been incredibly uplifting and satisfying. He finally realized his dream of producing safe, effective, and simple cures for the body and mind. At the same time, it must have also been a great relief as the last six months had been a great strain on him, and he needed to take some time to recover.

He carried on seeing patients, and by this time his sensitivity had become so acute that he would often develop the symptoms of his next patient before they arrived.

The Last Summer

In the summer of the following year, he wrote *The Twelve Healers and Other Remedies,* a book that is the cornerstone of this system of healing. It makes the remedies and the process of prescribing clear and simple to understand, qualities that Dr. Bach himself wanted to communicate to others. He gave the first of a series of lectures called "The Healing Herbs" on September 24, 1936, his fiftieth birthday, with the intention of sharing the discovery of the remedies with as many people as possible.

Toward the end of October 1936, he became ill and was confined to bed, but he still continued to work with the help of his assistants. His health improved for a short time, but then on the night of November 27, 1936, he died peacefully in his sleep. Toward the end of his life, shortly after discovering the last remedies, Dr. Bach said to a close friend, "I have nearly completed my work, I won't be with you much longer."

Dr. Bach's legacy to humankind cannot be quantified or described in words. His thoughts and actions were always directed toward the welfare of others. Within one short lifetime, he accomplished a work of great genius and love, the future results of which will be his greatest epitaph. Dr. Bach's wish that as many people as possible should benefit from this system of medicine is now being fulfilled as a result of the tireless efforts of those at the Bach Flower Centre at Mount Vernon. The current worldwide popularity of the remedies has come about mainly through word of mouth and Dr. Bach's own small advertisement in *The Northern Daily Telegraph* in 1932.

We often think of Dr. Bach working alone in his search to find the remedies, and this is true up to a point. He did receive much assistance from two people in particular: Nora Weeks and Victor Bullen. As mentioned earlier, Nora was a constant and supportive companion. They first met when Nora was working as a radiographer for one of Dr. Bach's medical colleagues.

They had a lot in common and became good friends. Nora recognized that Dr. Bach had special qualities over and above those of a typical doctor, and she was always interested to hear about his research and findings. When Dr. Bach decided to leave London and devote all his time to developing his new theories, he asked Nora to come and work with him as his assistant; she did not hesitate.

They spent much time together sharing their thoughts and ideas, and Nora often accompanied Dr. Bach on his long walks to find new remedies. Later on in Cromer, Victor Bullen, a local builder, became an important part of the team, helping out in whatever way he could. It was Nora who found Mount Vernon and the little cottage, which became Dr. Bach's beloved home and where he did so much of his work on the final nineteen remedies. Dr. Bach was very happy living at Mount Vernon. He loved gardening and walking in the surrounding countryside, and many of the flowers and trees he used to prepare the remedies can be found growing around and about the area, even in his garden.

In time, Nora and Victor became very skilled in prescribing the Bach Flower Remedies, and they continued to practice and share this knowledge with as many people as possible long after Dr. Bach had died. Their successors were John Ramsell and Nickie Murray. The Bach Centre is now run by John Ramsell and his daughter, Judy Howard, along with a number of helpers. Without the hard work of Dr. Bach's successors, it is possible that the purity and clarity of his work could have been lost.

Before Dr. Bach died, he told Nora and Victor that the Bach remedies would become the "medicine of the future," and that their use would spread throughout the world. He also said that distortions would arise and that many people would want to change the remedies and try to improve on them. He wanted people to know that the Bach remedies formed a complete system of healing by itself, and that a good knowledge of human nature was all that was required to become proficient in their use.

Thanks to his predictions, warnings, and advice not to change the remedies in any way, as well as the devotion of Dr. Bach's successors, the remedies have lost none of their potency. The remedies produced by the Bach Centre that we use today are identical to those that Dr. Edward Bach first discovered and prepared with his own hands.

Three

Reflections on Dr. Bach's Life

Dr. Bach's wish to help others surfaced in many ways throughout his life. From the time he left London to the end of his life, he never charged any fees for his work. He believed that good health was a birthright and should be freely available to all. He also strongly believed that all he would ever need would come naturally if he had faith and a good heart. This was just the case. He always had just enough resources to continue his work. Often the money he needed was received through contributions and gifts, and many people were always willing to help him. He was a natural giver in many ways; he always took an active role in community life when in Cromer and the village of Sotwell where Mount Vernon is located. He never turned a patient away and was always willing to lend a hand in whatever way he could.

Perhaps what made Dr. Bach special, what gave him his drive and ambition to fulfill his life's purpose, was the degree to which he thought about the welfare of others. Most of us are mainly concerned about our own happiness and the happiness of those closest to us. In fact, we never forget about our own happiness, even in our dreams. All our daily actions are generally motivated by this personal search for happiness. Dr. Bach realized that this way of thinking and living is what actually causes a lot of our problems. There is a special and lasting peace, happiness, and contentment to be found in the practice of cherishing others more than ourselves. Dr. Bach taught this by example.

If we concentrate on satisfying only our own needs for happiness, we will never achieve this goal—it is impossible. This selfishness, if allowed to continue and deepen, can easily become mentally and physically destructive to one's self and others. By always looking inward and only thinking about our own welfare, our mind becomes like an infinitely deep black hole that can never be filled. However, if we gradually try to seek happiness by helping others to be happy, we will never be separated from a happy mind. This, of course, does not mean that we should be hard on ourselves, give all our possessions away, or give all our time and energy to others. This would only be another extreme. We have to exercise our mind of cherishing others with wisdom. Cherishing others is primarily a state mind and a way of being. Externally our actions do not necessarily have to change as long as they are not harming others, while internally we are developing a consistent wish or intention to cherish others as much or more than we do ourselves. This is a special path to great happiness that Buddha, Jesus, and many great spiritual teachers taught.

Dr. Bach's external expression of this inner path was his devotion to a life of helping the sick. However, without his inner wish to help others and the sense of great happiness and fulfillment it brought him, he would not have been motivated to help others externally and we would not now have the Bach Flower Remedies. This inner wish or attitude toward others is what makes a great healer.

Buddha said that "illness has many good qualities." This is true if we can transform what we cannot cure into the path to inner happiness. Often illness dispels pride and helps us develop such qualities as patience and contentment. Serious illness really concentrates the mind. It can certainly make us think more deeply about what we value in life and help us reassess our priorities, attitudes, and lifestyle. Of course, no one would recommend "learning from illness" as a path, but there are so many examples of people whose lives have been positively transformed simply by learning to look at themselves and their lives in a new light.

Illness is not necessarily a negative force; in fact, it can be just the opposite. Simply by changing our mind, we can transform illness or any adverse condition into a meaningful opportunity to develop our own inner qualities. We never know what life is going to throw at us, but we can be ready for it if we are flexible, positive, and willing to accept difficulties and use them to become more whole and healthy human beings.

This raises the question: What is good health? Is it a healthy body or a healthy mind? Many New Age thinkers would say that it is a balance between the two, but if we analyze this, we can see that good health is simply a state of mind. Some people have developed the capacity to be deeply happy and content in the most adverse situations. Dealing with great physical or environmental difficulties and becoming stronger, more whole, and complete human beings because of it, those people have often become spiritually and mentally healthy. Certainly our inner achievements are ultimately of more value than our external triumphs.

So often the simple antidote to potential illness is to stop and think before illness makes you stop and think. Regularly giving yourself time to look at your life and the way you are living it is really important. Regular meditation, prayer, walks outdoors, or whatever helps you to get in touch with yourself and develop a little wisdom and clarity is priceless. It helps us to see where we are going and what might be coming in the future. It is not as difficult to see into the future as we think. It is simply a task of knowing that if we do not change our way of living, then the past will tend to repeat itself and the future is generally a simple projection of the present.

Being happy is an art that most of us have forgotten, yet it is not difficult to find happiness within when someone points us in the right direction. Developing inner happiness and contentment is a great treasure that we can all have in abundance simply by understanding and changing our inner nature. Understanding the true causes of happiness and suffering is right at the heart of Buddhist philosophy. (If you are interested in knowing more about Buddhism, refer to appendix 1.)

In fact, all we really need is a happy mind. Dr. Bach was a great example of this. He led his life in a very natural and simple way. He never felt that life owed him anything; he was a natural giver. He never needed much, and what he did have he either gave away or used with others in mind. He was simply very happy and that was all he needed.

At the end of his life, when he felt that he had done all he could to help others, he died with a happy and contented mind. By never wishing for his own happiness he found everlasting happiness. While Dr. Bach was a devout Christian, he thought in a very Buddhist way. His approach to life and his concern for the welfare of others showed great wisdom and compassion. We know that he had some understanding of the Buddhist path and deeply appreciated the wisdom of Buddha's teachings. In fact, he mentions the Buddha twice in his seminal text, *Heal Thyself,* once at the beginning and once at the end:

Five hundred years before Christ some physicians of ancient India, working under the influence of the Lord Buddha, advanced the art of healing to so perfect a state that they were able to abolish surgery, although the surgery of their time was as efficient, or more so, than that of the present day. (p. 7)

In our Western civilization we have the glorious example, the great standard of perfection and the teachings of the Christ to guide us. . . . Thus also taught the Buddha and other great masters who have come down from time to time upon the Earth to point out the way to attain perfection. There is no halfway path for humanity. The truth must be acknowledged. . . . (p. 56)

The word "Buddha" simply means "awakened one." Dr. Bach understood this concept. It was his aim to help people understand and walk such a path of self-awareness for the benefit of others. The best way we can help others is by becoming all that we can be ourselves. To do this, we need to know ourselves intimately, to know our own mind, and realize our own true nature—our greatest potential for good. This may sound like an impossible task or some dreamy solution to very real problems in the world, but it is actually a very simple and natural process that many are practicing and gaining practical benefits from. By learning to understand our mind, realizing and making the most of our positive inner qualities, we can solve our daily problems and find genuine and lasting peace, happiness, and contentment. Then if we wish, we can help others to gain the same freedom from suffering.

We cannot buy these inner qualities, yet they are of the highest value. We have to make an effort to develop them and keep them. This can be achieved most easily if we are walking a spiritual path or path to personal growth that is sincere, complete, tried, and tested. If we try to succeed alone or if we choose a path that is not genuine, we might progress but eventually slip back into our old patterns of negativity and self-doubt. Having someone special to guide and support your progress along with others to compare notes and share the journey with is a great help and a guarantee of success.

If we are spiritually poor, we have nothing to give, and we often feel that the world and those around us owe us much. This miserly or selfish mind causes lots of problems in our relationships, our health, and our general peace of mind. Making a decision to find a spiritual path that has clarity and meaning is a brave one, especially if it means having to change our lifestyle and give up some of our old beliefs and bad habits.

The special human qualities that Dr. Bach displayed and the story of his life are a great benchmark by which we can measure our own progress toward self-improvement. They are also a great example of what we can achieve in our life if we have a good heart and a strong will to succeed. There are many lessons we can learn from Dr. Bach's story, and we can gain much guidance in our use and understanding of the Bach Flower Remedies simply by studying them and trying to connect with the special inner qualities that Dr. Bach epitomized.

Four

How the Bach Remedies Work

Buddhism has, at its heart, the wisdom of understanding the mind. By examining this, we can gain insight into how the Bach remedies actually work and how we can use them effectively.

The Bach remedies represent the highest, most positive, and altruistic of human qualities. Although they were originally conceived to cure illness, they can also be used to develop whatever positive qualities we may be lacking. In fact, the Bach remedies can be a great support to spiritual development and personal growth. If we believe that all illnesses have their roots in the mind, as Dr. Bach did, we could also say that using the remedies is a form of preventative medicine. In fact, we can regard all our positive thoughts, words, and deeds as preventative medicine.

The remedies can help us develop positive qualities and abandon negative attitudes. In the short run, positive thoughts and emotions create a sense of contentment and well-being. In the long run, if we believe that what we "put out" into the world eventually comes back to us, then we are also investing in a healthy and happy future.

Through his early studies and research, Dr. Bach became aware that to find a truly effective form of healing that would strike at the root of ill-health, he would have to understand the true causes of illness. This led him in a similar direction as Samuel Hahnemann and to the idea that the true cause and cure of disease is not simply a physical phenomena but psychological in origin. The physical symptoms of disease are simply an external manifestation of inner "dis-ease." Given the fact that they both had little knowledge of psychology, Dr. Bach and Hahnemann were still able to deduce that successful remedies would have to work on the mental origins of the malady to effect a lasting cure.

Dr. Bach knew that he would have to discover remedies that would work on the subtle mental and emotional levels of the mind. He would have to find remedies that were able to dispel negative states of mind and promote positive ones. These remedies would have to be specific enough to target the particular negative states of mind that were giving rise to the physical symptoms. He realized that if the patient's state of mind could be improved when the appropriate remedy was prescribed, this would lead to improved physical health. He also realized that homeopathic remedies in general carried some form of healing energy or life force that directly improved the patient's frame of mind and physical health.

Dr. Bach and Hahnemann were men of great wisdom, and their discoveries and philosophies were way ahead of their time and still way ahead of modern psychology and medicine. Both their systems achieved incredible results and brought great benefit to countless people. However, without the skills required to fully understand the mind, they were unable to explain exactly how the remedies worked and to what extent they would prevent future illnesses. For answers to these questions, we have to look to a source of wisdom that is unparalleled.

If Dr. Bach had been able to study Buddhism in more depth, he would have discovered a wealth of information relating to life force energy and how this affects physical and mental health. This is a fascinating and in-depth subject that holds many answers to the questions that modern-day healers and therapists are asking: how does healing work, what are healing energies, where do they come from, and how do they actually work to improve health.

Life Force Energy

Although most people cannot see it, modern physics tells us that beyond the level of the smallest particles of matter, energy exists everywhere—in the air we breathe, in our food and water, and in the light from the sun.

Even inanimate objects possess a low or slow frequency of energy.

We could say that life force energy is the subtle foundation of all life. It supports, nourishes, and sustains the constant cycle of birth, life, and death. When we are in touch with this energy through prayer, meditation, or the Bach remedies, we feel less "separate" and increasingly "whole" within ourselves and within the whole of creation. We experience a sense of unity, we become more aware of our place or role in the great scheme of things, and at the same time we feel supported, safe, open, and confident. This in turn has a corresponding effect on our health, and if we continue to encourage and develop this special relationship with our higher nature, it also helps to prevent future illness. It's really just about being all that we can be and being happy with that.

From Buddhism and other Eastern spiritual traditions, we know that there are two main types of life force energy: internal and external. Internal life force energy is the subtle energy that exists within the body and mind of all living beings. External life force energy exists within plants, flowers, trees, rocks, minerals, crystals, etc. This energy is often harnessed for healing purposes as in the Bach Flower Remedies, crystal healing, flower essences, and homeopathic and herbal remedies. Spiritual and Reiki healers also channel a pure form of this energy and transfer it to the person they are healing.

A walk in the countryside or by the sea can also have a calming and healing effect on the body and mind. There is so much pure external life force energy available in these places that it "lifts" our own internal energies, creating positive effects on our body and mind. Conversely, if we spend too much time in urban areas or stressful environments where natural energies are restricted, this may adversely affect our health, especially if we are unable to transform or "rise above" these situations. Dr. Bach always felt happier and more relaxed when he was out of the city and enjoying the peace and openness of the countryside. He was obviously very sensitive to energy due to his abilities to diagnose problems easily and quickly. However, he himself became weak and fell ill easily if his own energy was depleted or degraded by being in the city.

Internal life force energy (sometimes called "chi" or "ki") runs through subtle channels or meridians in the human body. When these are blocked or unbalanced, due to stress, for example, illness can result. Most complementary therapies seek to help the body and mind rebalance and cleanse these internal energies, thereby promoting health and well being. This is also how the Bach remedies work as a healing technique. They are simple, pure, gentle, and effective healing agents.

There are many levels of internal and external life force energy in the universe. On one level, the Bach remedies are a very pure form of external life force energy. They can have a profound effect on our health and well-being by rebalancing, cleansing, and renewing our internal energy system. When the pure life force energy held within the remedy comes into contact with the internal life force energy of a human or animal that is blocked, sluggish, or unbalanced, it naturally and effort-lessly dissolves, "transmutes," and raises the quality of that energy to the healthiest level that the body, mind, and environment allows.

Conscious Energy

The only difference between internal and external energy is that internal life force energy has consciousness or "mind" and cannot exist separately from it. Due to the close relationship between consciousness and internal life force energy, it is easy to believe that the sense of close-ness or companionship we feel toward trees, crystals, the earth, or other sources of external life force energy is because they possess a personal character or mind. Exter-nal life force energy, like that within trees, crystals, and the earth, does not possess consciousness or mind. How-ever, this does not make them any less special or sacred "living" objects.

Our internal energies and our mind are inseparable; they exist almost as one and have a very intimate, dependent relationship. In fact, although we do not generally notice it, our thoughts and feelings "ride" on our internal energies. If we carry positive internal life force energy of a good quality, perhaps even enhanced by the Bach remedies, it is easier for us to develop posi-tive states of mind. Then we can attract positive life experiences and deal with problems more easily. Like-wise, if we consciously try to develop positive states of mind, like confidence, kindness, and wisdom, this will raise the quality of our internal energies and in turn improve our health and many other aspects of our life.

We can see, then, that with good motivation, the Bach remedies can assist us in improving our quality of life, helping us become more whole and healthy on many levels.

When internal and external life force energy are in harmony, possessing the same level of purity, existing on the same frequency, and within the same realm of existence, they are very similar energies. This is how external life force energy in the form of the Bach Flower Remedies is able to heal the mind and body. Each Bach remedy holds a specific type or level of external life force energy, vibrating at a certain frequency that directly corresponds to, or is the direct antidote to, a negative internal life force energy that is supporting a negative state of mind. When the internal energy system is consistently flooded with this positive external life force energy by taking the appropriate remedy, it completely cleanses and washes away the negative internal energies. It is then impossible for the negative state of mind to continue as there is no negative energy for it to "ride" on. It is also much easier for positive states of mind to arise as there is so much positive energy available.

As physical illness is directly related to the quality of our internal energies, the predominant negative state of mind that accompanies an illness is really a symptom of the negative internal energy that is creating the conditions for the illness to manifest. We cannot say that the negative state of mind is the cause of the illness. If this were true, then everyone with a particular negative state of mind would develop the same illness or at least some kind of illness, and everyone with a very positive state of mind would never be ill. This is obviously not the case. We could say that along with poor quality internal energies, negative minds are a condition that encourage illness to arise but, as explained later, we need to look deeper within the nature of the mind to discover the actual cause of illness.

Healthy Mind, Healthy Body

To cure an illness, the appropriate Bach remedy is prescribed by looking at the mental and emotional symptoms—not the physical ones. This tells us what type of negative internal energy needs to be replaced by the correct external life force energy remedy. Because of the close dependent relationship of our internal energies and our mind, we can say that each directly affects the other. Positive states of mind encourage and create healthy internal energies and vice versa. As physical health is directly related to the quality of our internal energies, therefore it is also directly affected by our thoughts and emotions.

We can prove this by simple logical reasoning. Some people can remain perfectly happy and content while experiencing poor health and even in the face of death when the internal energies that create good health have become weak and impure. Plants and trees can also develop diseases and die resulting from poor internal energies, and they have no mind or consciousness. This shows that life force energy has a direct influence on health, but that the accompanying mind, although not a cause of illness, can have an influence on it by prolonging or shortening an illness or by influencing its severity. There is much evidence to support this. For example, we know that the immune system is directly affected by a person's state of mind and that people with a long-term illness stand a much better chance of improving if they have a positive outlook. This mental influence is greatly increased if we can use our mind to consciously improve our internal energies through positive thinking and meditation. What actually causes poor quality energy to arise and create illness will be examined later when we look at the laws of karma, the root cause of all problems and good fortune.

When someone is successfully treated with a Bach remedy, the effect of the correct dose of positive external life force energy is the removal or transformation of the negative internal energy that is replaced with positive external energy. This is so like the natural positive internal energies that should be there that the body and mind immediately accepts them and reacts in a completely positive and natural way. After an appropriate length of treatment, the positive energy that is required to facilitate a complete and long-term cure arises naturally. In effect, the remedies create the opposite of dependence and actually encourage and remind the mind what energy it should be creating or allowing to arise naturally to ensure good mental and physical health. The remedies remind us how to create and maintain good health. Of course, all this is going on at a very subtle level within the body and mind so the process feels very natural, and we are usually not aware of what is actually happening within, as most people have little awareness of their own subtle or subconscious mind. The initial external manifestations of this process are increased vitality and peace of mind, a sense of well-being, and a more positive outlook accompanied by the first signs of physical improvement. Dr. Bach said that one of the most common remarks from a patient who was responding well to treatment was, "I feel more like myself again." This feeling is a good indication that the healing process is progressing well, even if no physical improvements have become apparent as yet.

The way in which the various internal energies, or subtle winds as they are called in Buddhism, affect and control physical and mental health is a very detailed area of study. There are Buddhist texts available that fully explain this fascinating subject (see "Further Reading"), however, a detailed knowledge is not necessary to be a good Bach flower therapist. Dr. Bach himself had little knowledge of this area and showed that all we need to make the most of the remedies is a little understanding of human nature, which we all have, and a strong wish to help others. In fact, the power of our compassion is the most potent remedy we possess.

So it would seem there are many facets to the Bach Flower Remedies. They are not just simple healing remedies. Many people from both religious and nonreligious backgrounds have noticed their spiritual lives renewed or reborn as a result of the Bach remedies, almost as if they have the ability to lead people, if they wish, to a deeper awareness of their own spirituality or potential for personal growth. When our internal energies are pure, our mind is pure. Each of the remedies carries an energy that encourages and supports positive, nonselfish states of mind and, if we use the correct remedies regularly, we will naturally want to improve ourselves and help others. We can use the remedies to help us achieve this altruistic and healthy outlook. We could not say that the remedies possess wisdom or any conscious qualities, because, as explained earlier, external life force energy is just energy. However, they are closely related to consciousness because the high vibrational quality of each remedy is similar to the subtle energy that our mind require to function. We know that external energy can appear to exist without mind, but that mind or consciousness cannot exist without internal energy and vice versa. Negative minds need negative energy to exist, so if we can raise the quality of our internal life force energy by using the Bach remedies or any other pure source of life force energy or blessing, then we can really begin to enjoy a more healthy, fulfilling, and meaningful life. We can move closer to our natural potential for good.

There are many paths to personal and spiritual growth nowadays, and it seems that most of them are pointing in a similar direction. This would suggest most paths eventually lead into one, and that one true path leads to one source, and that source is emanating these paths according to our individual needs and tendencies. So perhaps in this way we can see the remedies as an expression of a supreme level of consciousness whose essence is complete wisdom and compassion. If we know that consciousness "rides" on internal life force energy, then perhaps we can see the remedies as a connection to the universal internal life force energy of the most open, advanced, expanded, and pure form of consciousness. The remedies may just presently appear to us as simply external energy because of our current lack of deep insight and limited awareness. The remedies certainly represent the selfless qualities that all of the great spiritual teachers of the past and present have shown and taught, such as wisdom, love, compassion, patience, joyous effort, and steadfastness.

Many people who are sensitive to energy feel a spiral of energy coming from above, down through the head or crown chakra, and into the mind and body when they take the remedies. This experience is similar to receiving spiritual healing, Reiki healing, or receiving blessings from above when praying or meditating. Often for a few minutes after taking the remedy, sometimes longer, some people feel a cushion of energy surrounding the body, and the mind becomes quite peaceful. Disturbing thoughts and worries subside, and there is a sense of physical relaxation as tension is released. So again, this would suggest that the remedies connect us to the source of some kind of spiritual blessing. Whether we call this source God, Buddha, Allah, or our own higher nature is not too important. What is important is that we reach out to connect with it in a way that feels comfortable and natural to us. This may be through prayer, meditation, by taking a walk in the country, whatever brings us back to ourselves and leaves us feeling more whole and complete, relaxed, content, blessed, and protected. We need this to live. As Dr. Bach taught, it is as vital to our health and well-being as clean air and good food.

If we consciously and regularly seek this inner communion, we will find a constant and unwavering source of peace and happiness that is a refuge against the changing fortunes of life. Spending time in this way may initially seem selfish, but if by doing this we are more able to help others, then it can be quite a selfless act, especially if helping others is our main motivation in the first place. This practice of inner growth can also be a great support to the healing process itself, especially if we use the Bach remedies to overcome some mental or physical problems.

Many Buddhist texts refer to life force energy as subtle wind. This is a good description of how many people experience the remedies. We could refer to the remedies as a pure subtle wind or blessing coming from a special place, perhaps "pure wind from a pure land." "Pure land" is the Buddhist term for "heaven," an outward manifestation of the mind of enlightenment.

As limited beings, we live in a world of conflicting conceptual thought or duality: good and bad, light and dark, internal and external, have and have not, self and other. The healing "essence" of the remedies seems to transcend and go beyond the duality of an internal or external world toward a balanced completeness, unity, and wholeness, where there are no limitations of identity or barriers between the self and others. Perhaps, ultimately, this essence is inexpressible or indescribable, only experiential, boundless loving kindness, wisdom, beauty, and perfection.

Many spiritual traditions honor the idea of full enlightenment; indeed, as mentioned, the word "Buddha" means "Awakened One." The mind of enlightenment pervades the whole of space and time and perceives the true nature of all phenomena directly and simultaneously. It is the syntheses of the greatest peace, joy, love, compassion, and wisdom. Buddha's main purpose or intention is to relieve and prevent suffering and bring all living beings to the same state of complete consciousness or wholeness, if that is what they wish. Many followers of other religions would also equate this idea with their own perception of God. Perhaps then the gift of the Bach Flower Remedies as a healing technique is an expression or emanation of this loving kindness, a form of blessing, empowerment, and connection to a higher source that is very close to our own true nature and has our own best intentions at heart.

Creating Your Own Reality

We all live in a slightly different universe. Animals experience a different world than humans, but every human also experiences the outside world in a different way. We each have different perceptions of the same things caused by having different mind sets, and these perceptions can change over time. For example, when we are young we may not like curry, but as we grow older we may change our mind and stop perceiving curry as a source of displeasure. Instead, we may actually begin to see curry as a source of pleasure. Curry did not change; it was never inherently good or bad. We can apply this to any phenomena. Nothing is inherently good or bad; we project these qualities onto objects, people, and places and believe them to be real. Another good example is when we meet someone for the first time. We immediately form an opinion of them; however, that first opinion is often proved to be wrong, and we may easily grow to like or dislike that person given time.

So what relevance does this have to the Bach remedies? Well, simply this:

Peaceful mind = peaceful world.

The remedies help us change our mind; not the world around us, but by changing our mind, all things change. Our perception of ourself, our environment, and others changes completely when we change our mind or when our mind is changed. This tried and tested ancient wisdom for solving all our problems can be summed up in one phrase:

All we need is a happy mind.

We will never find lasting happiness by trying to manufacture a perfect world for ourselves. We can try to find the best job, the right partner, the nicest house, or the fastest car and, for a short time, we may find some happiness in these things. If we are honest, we know in our heart that this happiness will come to an end. It is not real happiness and often serves to create more problems than it solves. In fact, the amount of pain and unhappiness we experience when we are separated from these things will at the very least be proportionate to the amount of attachment we have to them. There is a strong relationship between need and pain. The more we need someone or something to make us happy, the more pain we will experience when we are eventually parted from them.

We also spend much time and effort manipulating our world to get what we want, when we want it, but all the happiness and peace of mind we could wish for is literally under our nose. If we have a happy mind, we can experience all manner of difficult circumstances and unpleasant situations and not feel any less happier. We also know that if we are deeply unhappy, no amount of money, possessions, or relationships can help us. Again, this shows that happiness depends on the mind, not on external factors. Understanding this simple wisdom and taking it to heart should give us great hope, because it is the root of all spiritual attainments:

The door of the mind is the gateway to heaven.

Learning to open our heart and mind and develop some simple wisdom and contentment is time well spent, and the rewards for accumulating these inner treasures are fathomless. This is not some difficult or mystical task. It is very simple and natural to all of us, and we can use the Bach remedies to help us begin and complete this journey toward great lasting happiness.

To walk a path of spiritual or personal growth does not mean we have to shave our head and run to the hills. This would be another extreme and another way of trying to manipulate the world to avoid what we dislike. Real spiritual practitioners realize that they have exactly the right conditions at present to start developing higher qualities within themselves. Whether we are rich or poor does not matter; what matters is that we make an effort to change from within. Simply by making a daily determination to be a little more tolerant, patient, kind, and helpful is a great step forward. Then if we can carry forward these determinations into our daily activities and remind ourself of our good intentions, especially when we are challenged by our own impatience or selfishness, then we will begin to make real progress.

Again, we can change our inner qualities simply by changing our mind. We are not inherently good or bad people. We have just developed mental habits one way or the other, and these mental habits can be changed, some quickly, some slowly. Getting to know and regularly using the Bach remedies is a great aid to this process of inner healing.

The Bach Flower Remedies work in two ways: they heal existing problems and prevent future ones from arising. They do this by preventing the potential causes of illness from arising deep within the mind. Illness can only arise from within the mind if the right conditions are present. For example, a seed cannot grow into a tree without water, soil, light, and air. Likewise a potential illness will find it difficult to arise if we eliminate stress, a poor diet, a depressing environment, and, most importantly, negative states of mind and poor quality internal energies. Using the Bach remedies is protection against these conditions.

From Buddhism we know that any illness, before manifesting on the physical or conscious level, initially arises from the subtle or deepest levels of the mind, which are subconscious to most people. Ultimately, we can only remove the true causes of illness by knowing, experiencing, and purifying our subtle mind of all potential "seeds" of illness planted or created by our past negative actions in previous lives. This is our karma. Even when these seeds ripen or are removed, the mental imprints of these past actions still remain, like footprints in the sand. These create the mental tendencies to walk the same path again or commit similar negative actions in the future. These imprints must also be removed if we want to fully prevent illness or other negative experiences in this life and future lives. One way we can do this is by completely purifying our subtle mind and developing a special type of wisdom through practicing certain simple meditation techniques taught in Buddhism (see appendix 1).

Karma — Actions and Their Effects

Basically, we can say that any disease, disorder, or unhappiness is the result of some disharmony in the body, mind, or environment. However, it is not an easy task to establish the original cause of a particular problem. From Buddhism we know that the root causes of all our major and minor problems are our own previous negative actions of body, speech, and mind returning to us as illness, poverty, ignorance, or any other unpleasant experience. The word "karma" directly translates as "action," or what we intentionally create mentally, verbally, or physically. The laws of karma teach that whatever we create or give out comes back to us sooner or later, just like a boomerang. These negative actions may have been performed many lifetimes ago, and it is only now that we might be experiencing the repercussions. We may think that we would never have committed serious negative actions like harming others, but our previous lives are almost completely different from the life we are living now. If we met ourselves from a previous life, we would not recognize ourselves at all. It would be like meeting a complete stranger.

Buddhism suggests that each lifetime we are almost born anew. On the surface we all have completely different bodies and personalities, yet deep within our subtle mind, soul, or higher self we carry the memories, tendencies, and imprints of all our previous lives. When the conditions are right, our previous actions will return to us as positive or negative experiences, depending on whether they were well intentioned, beneficial, or otherwise. So from a Buddhist perspective, to fully heal and prevent future illness, we must remove the root causes, or seeds, of our past negative actions from deep within the mind before they ripen as unpleasant experiences.

Dr. Bach knew about karma, and he had a strong interest in all religions and philosophies. In *Heal Thyself* he says:

> *Man's body is himself externalized, an objective manifestation of his internal nature. . . . The materialization of the qualities of his consciousness.*
> (p. 56)

We could just as easily say that any man is simply the result of his previous actions ripening as pleasant or unpleasant characteristics and experiences. However, because one person is experiencing happiness and good fortune does not necessarily mean they are superior than others or that they have been kinder or more giving in previous lives. We all have an infinite amount of accumulated karma, because we have had countless previous lives. We have all been good and bad people in previous lives, so we don't know what karma will ripen next—it might be pleasant, it might not. Unfortunately, karma ripens haphazardly; there is no grand plan or great scheme. Life is simply a "karmic lottery." If the conditions are right, any sort of karma could ripen, anything could happen to us. A murderer can be reborn as a king in his next life if he has the right karma from a previous life. He may experience many fortunate rebirths in wealthy and loving families until eventually the karma of his murderous life catches up with him.

We can protect ourselves from our own karma by completely purifying it while we have the wisdom and opportunity to do so. We cannot escape the law of karma simply by not believing it. According to many religions and philosophies, it is a fact of life, and we have to face that. Dr. Bach said:

> *The abolition of disease will depend upon human-ity realizing the unalterable laws of our universe and adapting itself with humility and obedience to those laws. . . .* (p. 40)

Sometimes no matter how hard we try and no matter what therapies or remedies we use, we cannot escape or remove the effects of heavy negative karma that might be ripening in the form of a serious and possibly life-threatening illness. Of course, we can use the Bach remedies to help us deal with such challenging situations, but we also have to be realistic. Sometimes we simply have to accept what is happening to us and stop fighting. Developing a peaceful and happy mind is possible even in the face of great hardship. Learning to accept the things we cannot change and developing compassion for others who may be feeling sadness shows great wisdom and maturity. Accepting difficulties with a peaceful and patient mind actually purifies the effects of negative karma and exhausts it much more quickly than if we develop anger or sadness.

Selfishness—The Source of All Suffering

The main cause of illness is negative karma ripening when the conditions are favorable. But what causes us to create negative karma? The simple answer is our selfish mind. Likewise a selfless mind can cause us to create positive karma that will come back to us as a pleasant experience in the future. Why was Dr. Bach so naturally compassionate, courageous, and wise? Perhaps because he had made great efforts to develop those qualities in previous lives and, as a result of that, those qualities were arising naturally and spontaneously within him. Dr. Bach says in *Heal Thyself* that:

> *The cause of all our troubles is self and separateness and this vanishes as soon as love . . . becomes part of our nature.* (p. 55)

In other words, thinking of the welfare of others is a great source of future happiness, and thinking of our own welfare is a source of future suffering. Even in the short term, transferring our attention toward others and working for their benefit can take our mind off our own problems and cause us to be less introverted and self-obsessed. The more we worry about a problem, the bigger it gets, but the more we concern ourselves with helping others, the less energy and time we give to our own worries, and the weaker and less demanding they become.

We can use this line of reasoning in many practical ways. For example, if we have to give a public speech, we may be anxious or frightened, especially if we have little experience. We should then think about how we can help these people. By strongly concentrating on these thoughts, our own worries will naturally diminish. This line of reasoning is powerful and can be applied to many situations that cause unhappiness or worry.

One of our greatest sources of happiness or unhappiness is relationships. Concentrating on the welfare of the other person in a relationship will definitely help us become more content and less demanding or controlling. All great spiritual teachers know that the source of all happiness is caring for others—all others equally. Again, Dr. Bach says:

> *Expect nothing from others, but, on the contrary be ever ready to lend a helping hand to lift them upwards in times of their need and difficulty.*
> (p.54)

The main factor in creating karma is our true intentions or motivations. Many people might appear to be altruistic and always doing good for others, but if their motivations are selfish, perhaps because they want others to like them, then this will not give rise to a good karmic "return" in the future. Conversely, leading a very normal life with pure motivation will lead to great future happiness.

We can say that illness arises from negative karma that was created by selfish actions in a previous life, but what causes us to perform selfish actions? What causes us to think and act in a selfish way? If we understand the answer to this, then we are truly on the way to solving all our problems and finding a lasting cure to any present or potential illness.

The Universal Cure

We act instinctively and naturally to benefit ourselves, because we think we are more important than others. Our sense of self is very dear to us and we cherish it deeply. We do not realize how deeply we cherish ourselves until we are faced with situations that frighten or challenge our sense of self; so we have a strong sense of self, a strong sense that we truly exist, and that this self is the most important thing in the universe. The fact that we grasp at this sense of self, ego, or I, and believe it to truly exist is the source of our present and future problems. If we could realize our true nature and abandon the ignorance that gives rise to the nonexistent self, we could solve all our problems and experience complete and lasting happiness and freedom from suffering forever.

We can compare the mind to a glass of sparkling water, with the constant stream of bubbles floating to the surface as our thoughts and feelings. It appears that we "are" these thoughts and emotions that arise from within, as if they make up our identity and character or as if they are the "real us." Our true nature is more like the water itself than the bubbles that arise in it. Our essence, or source, in reality, is closer to the space between our thoughts and feelings.

We cannot truly help others until we have healed ourselves, and a true healing is one that is complete and lasting and comes from within. We can only accomplish this by realizing our true nature and becoming all that we can be, then we will have the wisdom and power to help others achieve the same state of complete happiness and permanent freedom from unhappiness. To reach this destination, we have to find a clear and direct path.

Buddha taught such a path thousands of years ago. Many people realized his teachings then and found great happiness and inner peace as a result. Many people today are also finding this timeless wisdom invaluable and relevant to the problems they face. Buddhism is really "Truism." It simply tells us the way things are, the way things will be, and the way we can improve them.

Having said that, Buddhism does not have a monopoly on truth. Many of Buddha's teachings are reflected in all of the world's religions and spiritual paths to truth and happiness. We cannot say that one is superior or better than another. They all have good qualities, and perhaps we can say that they are all leading in a similar direction and come from the same source. As individuals, we have to find one that we feel comfortable with and one that we feel shines clarity and truth.

The Bach remedies can be a perfect accompaniment to following a path toward personal and spiritual growth. Dr. Bach realized that it was this path that was the universal cure and the most important aspect of being human. The remedies that arose from Dr. Bach's compassionate mind can help us develop the same qualities that he valued and taught as an inner path to happiness.

He himself said that if someone does not actually want to get well, then the remedies may not help them. They are of greatest effect when given to someone who is willing to make an effort to understand and improve themselves. In *Heal Thyself* Dr. Bach said:

> *Disease . . . will never be eradicated except by spiritual and mental effort. . . . if a patient knows or by some wise physician is instructed in the nature of the adverse spiritual or mental forces at work. . . . and if that patient attempts to neutralize those forces, health improves as soon as this is begun and when it is completed the disease will disappear. This is true healing by attacking the stronghold, the very base of the cause of suffering.*

If we can understand and improve ourselves, as Dr. Bach encouraged his patients to do, there can be no higher purpose to our life. Dr. Bach lived his life with great purpose and motivation. He strove to better himself and help others however he could, for he knew in his heart that when his inner qualities of compassion and wisdom finally became complete, he would be able to help countless living beings. In this way, he would realize his own true nature and actually become the universal cure for others.

Working toward and achieving our true nature is not a painful or monumental task. We all have the potential and the right conditions to achieve spiritual enlightenment. It is said that it is easier to gain enlightenment in one lifetime than it is to gain another human rebirth, so we have already done most of the work. We just need to make the most of the opportunity we now have.

Five

How to Prescribe the Remedies

Dr. Bach wanted to keep his new system of medicine as simple as possible so that anyone could use it with confidence. He did not leave any detailed instructions or complicated texts that would have to be studied before being able to use the remedies. The only text he wrote specifically about the remedies and how to use them is *The Twelve Healers and Other Remedies.* It is a small and easy-to-read booklet giving accurate but brief explanations of the thirty-eight remedies, when they should be used, and how to use them. It is invaluable to anyone wishing to make the most of the Bach remedies.

Dr. Bach destroyed many of his earlier notes and papers on the remedies, because it was his intention that people would only need brief, accurate details on how and when to use them. He did not want to complicate or confuse matters with theoretical or academic explanations.

Whatever mental, emotional, or physical condition we want to treat, all we have to do is identify those states of mind we or the person we are treating are experiencing and choose the appropriate remedies accordingly. We do not need to have knowledge of anatomy or physiology or be able to diagnose physical or mental illness, because we are not treating ourselves or others in this way. We only need to be able to recognize states of mind and simply ask others how they are feeling.

Of course, if we are treating others on a regular basis, we need to be sure that they are seeing a medical doctor if they have any serious conditions. We should never try to replace conventional treatments or medicines with the Bach remedies. The Bach remedies will work in harmony with any conventional therapy and will not cause adverse side effects. They are gentle healing agents without the possibility of overdose, addiction, or adverse effects from misdiagnosis. They are pure and natural remedies that contain little or none of the physical plant or tree, only the plant's healing life force energy held within the water and a little alcohol for preservation.

If we are diagnosing for ourselves or others, and we have some knowledge of the remedies, it is a simple task to choose the appropriate ones for use.

Steps for Prescribing

1. Conduct an interview to identify the states of mind that are present, i.e., anger, fear, indecision, anxiety, etc.

2. List all the remedies that are relevant to these states of mind. Determine the patient's type remedy.

3. Put them in order of severity or importance, keeping the list to within ten. This helps identify which remedies are most likely to be successful.

4. Choose the remedies we want to try from this list.

Remember, we are not treating a physical illness, so if someone has a strained ligament, for example, we should not choose Vervain because it is for people who tend to overexert themselves. Instead we need to establish what sort of person he or she is. What is the character and disposition of the person? How does he or she think and feel about him or herself and the world around them? For example, is the person dominant and controlling? Does he or she get angry easily? Is the person shy, or constantly distracted or dreamy? We need to have a good knowledge of the remedies to spot these mental traits, then we will begin to diagnose accurately and quickly.

There is no easy way to learn the remedies. Everyone has a different way of remembering things that works for them. A good way is to set a goal of remembering two or three remedies a day. Then within two or three weeks we will have a basic knowledge of all the remedies. Try to remember the key words at first (shown at the beginning of each remedy in chapter 8). When we have this basic knowledge we can begin to learn more about the remedies by using them as much as possible. The real key to success is developing the skill to recognize the relevant and predominant states of mind that someone is naturally disposed to or that accompany a particular illness.

Type Remedies

We all have a "type remedy." A type remedy is one, two, or sometime three remedies that make up the core or major traits of someone's personality. For example, it is easy to spot someone who is always impatient, quick in thought and action, and doesn't suffer fools gladly. This person's type remedy is Impatiens. People who are dreamy, as if in a world of their own, and tend to sleep a lot are classic Clematis types. It is interesting to begin spotting these traits in ourselves and others. We can learn a lot about human nature in this way, and we can do this kind of study anywhere, anytime, and no one has to know that we are practicing our diagnostic techniques.

Generally speaking, when we are prescribing a Bach remedy we should try to identify the type remedy and then add other remedies that are relevant for the short-term or easily changeable states of mind. For example, someone might be a Water Violet type—proud, aloof, quiet, a loner, intelligent, and artistic—but during illness he or she may have constant worries that go around and around in his or her head. This would then indicate White Chestnut. The solution is to use both remedies together, the White Chestnut being a more temporary remedy.

When choosing the final number of remedies, we should keep the number to within six or seven. Usually just one or two remedies are needed. Using too many remedies at once can confuse the picture, and we will not know which remedies are working and which are unnecessary. We need to use our own judgment and intuition, then with experience we will become skilled and accomplished healers.

Another good way of beginning our journey with the Bach remedies and also remembering them is to briefly read through the remedy descriptions and make a note of those that are relevant to our own personality and those people closest to us. Then we should buy those remedies and use them on ourselves and others. We might need a good friend to help us spot our own type remedy, someone who knows us well and is not afraid to be honest with us. Often we think we know ourselves well, but we can miss the traits that our subconscious selfish mind does not want us to admit. We are very good at spotting our good qualities but not so good at spotting our weaknesses. If we try this exercise with a friend who is also interested in the remedies, we can learn a lot about ourselves and the remedies while having fun, too.

After prescribing for ourselves and our friend, we should have a review session in two or three weeks to share our experiences. We may find that some remedies have gone straight to the heart of the matter, or we may decide to try others. Another useful idea is to keep a diary of our states of mind over a couple of weeks. Write down how we feel about ourself, our life, and how we react to certain situations. This can be a useful way to recognize predominant states of mind and those that are more fleeting and less deep-seated, then we can tailor our remedy accordingly.

If we are thinking of prescribing for others on a regular basis, it is a good idea to treat ourselves and those closest to us for a few months first and get to know the remedies well before going further.

Prescribing for Others

The key to successfully prescribing for others is simply learning to listen well. Let the other person guide the interview. Try not to be too intrusive; people are an open book if we know how to read them. Don't try too hard to pry them open. If they are shy and find it difficult to talk (Mimulus), or are obviously putting a brave face on things (Agrimony), these are immediate remedy indicators. If they talk too much about their own problems (Heather) this is also a big give-away. When we get to know the remedies well these personality traits will gradually become more obvious, and we will be able to spot them often within minutes of meeting someone.

It doesn't matter if we get the diagnosis wrong on the first or second attempts. All the Bach remedies have remarkable healing qualities, and even the wrong remedy can have good results. Sometimes in the pressure of an interview or therapy session we may not be able to think clearly enough to prescribe accurately. The best remedy may come to us later on when we are more relaxed and have had time to think about the interview. This is not a problem, simply include this remedy next time. If necessary, to be more relaxed and clear in thought during an interview, take the appropriate remedies beforehand, such as Mimulus for nervousness and Clematis for clearer thinking.

During the interview we may temporarily "pick-up" the patient's state of mind. For example, it might be a negative Clematis state that prevents us from thinking clearly. We don't need to experience this to make a good diagnosis. To guard against this, use the Walnut remedy, which can protect us from external influences. This is also a good remedy to use between therapy sessions to help us stay centered, strong, and clear.

If we intend to treat people on a regular basis, good counseling skills are very useful. Just learning to listen without judging is a special skill that is invaluable in the healing process. It creates an environment that helps the patient relax and feel more comfortable and able to talk openly about his or her problems. We can learn these skills from reading books, practicing on family or friends, or, preferably, taking a short course at a local college or center. Learning to listen also helps us develop our ability to tune in to others and their feelings, thoughts, and personal characteristics. Listening also helps us reduce our sense of self-importance, which increases our daily worries and problems and creates a mental barrier, preventing a clear and healthy client-therapist relationship. If we think other people are important, we are obviously going to treat them with respect and kindness.

The Bach remedies can be combined safely with any other type of alternative or complementary therapy. However, if we use them as Dr. Bach did, as a complete system of healing for mind and body, then we should regard them as a "nondirective" form of therapy. This means that we should try to let the client dictate which remedies are right for them by the simple diagnostic techniques outlined in this book, and then give the remedies time to work. Giving too much advice, no matter how well intentioned, can sometimes cause more problems than it solves, especially if the person being treated is feeling vulnerable. We can give verbal advice and guidance if the patient asks for it and if we feel strongly and clearly that it is appropriate.

The Healing Power of Compassion

What really makes for a good therapist or healer is a strong mind of compassion. From a Buddhist perspective, compassion is a mind that acts on the wish to relieve the suffering of others and to protect them from future suffering in the wisest way possible. This basic wish to benefit others is our "Buddha nature" and the source of many spiritual realizations. We could say that compassion is a wise action of body, speech, or mind that arises out of our empathy toward others. It is an empowering, active, and deeply fulfilling state of mind, and it is a long way from worry. Compassion is the opposite of, or the antidote to, worry. Worry is an uncomfortable, self-centered, inward-looking mind that restricts the free flow of healthy life force energy and brings more future problems. Compassion is a wide, outward-looking, giving, and deeply peaceful mind that creates a boundless and effortless flow of positive energy.

We can increase our compassion by regularly contemplating the difficulties and potential dangers that all living beings face, then firmly resolving to help them in whatever way we can. By doing this, we will eventually be able to directly release and protect others from suffering.

The best way to help others is by simply developing our own inner qualities of compassion and wisdom. Although externally it appears that these qualities are not very useful, as we develop them, we draw closer to our own greatest potential for good. Eventually, when we fully realize this potential, we will be able to benefit others in countless ways. If we need a little encouragement to begin this inner journey, it is worth considering that generating this wish and decision to help others, by walking a spiritual path, is the only way we will find true lasting happiness for ourselves.

Can the power of our compassion affect the Bach remedies that we prescribe for others? The simple answer is "Yes," but we may not be able to see this clearly. Again, the mind is a subtle object, and the effect of the thoughts and intentions that accompany our actions are not easily revealed unless we are familiar with our inner world. We can prove this in another way. If someone were to prescribe the Bach remedies, and he or she were in a very negative frame of mind, perhaps impatient or distracted and not that bothered about the welfare of the person he or she was treating, then this would obviously have a profound effect on the treatment. The client would sense this and not be at ease, leaving with little faith in the remedies. The therapist might also not choose the right remedies. Already many "doors" are closing and the chance of a successful treatment is reduced. Conversely, if the therapist has his or her client's best interests at heart and has a mind of great compassion, this will naturally lead to a successful treatment and also give the client confidence in the therapist and the treatment.

We also have to look again at karma to gain some clarity on this issue. The karma of the client and therapist is the key factor in the possibility of a successful treatment. There are two conditions that they can establish that will help the karma of a successful treatment to ripen. From the therapist's side, the mind of pure compassion is vital, and, from the patient's side, the minds of patience, faith, and the wish to be well are vital. Even if we only have a little of these qualities, that will give the remedies enough room to work well.

If patients can also develop more compassion for others, this will aid their own healing process. The opposite of compassion is a selfish mind, and selfish minds are one of the conditions that can encourage the karma of illness to ripen. Conversely, a wish to use our life well and help others whenever possible will help the karma of good health to ripen. It is important to stress that this is not a guarantee of good health. Many compassionate people suffer from illness. It is simply another condition that can influence health.

Whatever conditions we create, good and bad karma can only ripen if we have created the causes by planting the seeds of this karma by our actions of body, speech, and mind in previous lives. This is why some very negative people never get ill and have long lives and why some very positive people get ill and sometimes die young. It is all about causes and conditions. If we have not created the causes to be ill, or we have removed them through inner purification, whatever conditions we create, we will not become ill.

There is one more advantage in trying to develop our compassion. If selfish actions lead to future suffering, then compassion must lead to great health and happiness in the future.

There were occasions in Dr. Bach's life when he was able to heal simply through touch. This is relevant because, whenever it happened, he would have no warning but simply and naturally feel overwhelming compassion for his patient and feel the need to touch them. If the patient felt comfortable with this, he would feel a great surge of healing energy come through him from "above" and into the patient through his hands. A cure or relief from the illness would almost be immediate. The interesting point is that he would always feel this great sense of compassion first, and it would be this state of mind that created the bridge, channel, and environment for the healing energy to flow and ripen the patient's karmic seed of good health. This was not always possible because not many people have the karma to experience that kind of healing nowadays. However, the Bach remedies are so special because millions of people do have the karma to benefit from them today.

Transforming Illness into "The Path"

By using our mind and the Bach remedies, we can try to create the conditions that will give rise to good health. But what can we do when good health still does not arise? Hard times are never meaningless if we know how to transform them by using them to develop our inner qualities. From the point of view of dealing with illness, one of the most valuable qualities we can develop is patience and reduce our propensity for anger and frustration.

Often we see patience as being an uncomfortable "grit your teeth and bear it" state of mind. However, the truly patient mind is able to accept difficult circumstances while remaining peaceful and happy. Depending on our circumstances, this may not seem easy, especially as we so often feel justified in our judgement of others' wrong actions. No matter how justified we feel, if we check, anger or irritation is an uncomfortable mind. If we have been hurt by someone, why do we hurt ourselves more by feeling the pain of anger? We have a choice. Surely common sense tells us to develop the state of mind that will help the hurt heal sooner. If we burn our hand, we immediately put it under cold water, not hot. Developing anger can only be a cause of more conflict, whereas patience and understanding can actively diffuse confrontation and promote mutual understanding.

Patience does not mean that we should suppress anger, as this only leads to resentment, bitterness, and related physical illness in the future. Patience and forgiveness are the healing way between the extremes of either suppressing or indulging anger and other strong negative emotions. The practice of patience is a deeply transforming process. It creates a peaceful and stable mind and enables us to release negativity as it arises in the mind. Patience also gives us the mental space and clarity to judge our responses to challenging situations with wisdom, fairness, and honesty.

Practicing patience means willingly accepting and transforming everyday annoyances and difficulties into the path to personal happiness and inner contentment. Normally we would try to avoid any amount of irritation, but with gentle, consistent determination we can use these opportunities to gradually learn to relax, accept, and eventually welcome the chance to practice developing a peaceful mind in trying situations. Also in this way, we can quickly and directly purify the negative karma (previous negative actions) that are causing unpleasant circumstances to arise. Remembering this can help us maintain peaceful patience. This is actually the quickest way to purify negative karma that we are already experiencing, like illness, poverty, loneliness, and so on.

Anger can be the most damaging and destructive force known to humans. We should be ruthless with it and never allow ourselves to be controlled by it. When we are under the influence of anger, we easily lose control of our thoughts and actions, saying and doing things that we later regret. Just as a forest fire starts from one small spark, violent anger can easily develop in a mind that readily becomes frustrated or impatient with small problems. Anger gets us into trouble and pride keeps us there. Anger is our worst enemy. We should only ever get angry at our anger.

Buddha said: "Illness has many good qualities." There is no doubt that many people would disagree with this. How can any form of suffering be beneficial? We all work constantly to avoid suffering and to find happiness. However, the happiness we seek in the external world is transient and provides no lasting satisfaction. Often the temporary happiness we find in relationships and possessions only leads to greater unhappiness when we are parted from them. But the happiness that comes from a peaceful and content mind can never be stolen and will never leave us even when we die.

Many people develop such happiness by learning to live with illness and transform it into the inner path.

There are many instances of this happening. So what is the value of physical healing if it denies us the opportunity to develop such inner wisdom and happiness? Obviously we do not have to be ill to develop such qualities, but it can point us in the right direction. Then when we are familiar with that path and no longer need illness to point us in the right direction, that can be an appropriate time for healing. Again, there is no guarantee of this, but this is often what happens.

As a healer, the most important lesson to learn from all of this is that although we want people to be healthy, our main aim should be to help people make the most of the opportunities they have to find some lasting happiness now and in the future. This will only come about through realizing their own divinity or spiritual nature, not necessarily through good health and success in the external world. These are simple but challenging truths. Dr. Bach went out of his way to share this knowledge and wisdom with others. He was not simply and blindly bent on physical healing. If we read *Heal Thyself,* we will see that his real message to humanity was to look within for the answers.

One more interesting result of trying to develop our spiritual qualities is that we are able to enjoy our relationships and external possessions much more when we reduce our attachment and need for them. It is as if the less we need these things, the more fun we have. Having more space and clarity in our mind helps us to view the external world in a more playful way, while our regard for the really serious issues, like our wish for others to be happy, increases.

In conclusion, Dr. Bach taught by example that real freedom and happiness can be found simply by abandoning our selfish, needy mind and concentrating on helping others. If we strive to emulate this great man, our own practice and prescribing of the Bach remedies will become a powerful force for good.

Six

How to Prepare and Use the Remedies

Dr. Bach often said that nonmedically trained Bach flower practitioners were generally more accurate at prescribing than medical practitioners who often found it difficult to remove their attention from the physical illness. We know that the diagnostic aspect of this system of healing pays little regard to the physical aspects of the patient's problem, but to the predominant states of mind that indicate which remedies will have the most potent healing effect on the body and mind. With experience, we will notice that there are sometimes similarities between the physical complaints of people with the same type remedy, but this is not a rule, and we should never prescribe the remedies on this basis.

Choosing the right combination of remedies to suit the individual is the key to successful treatment. This might be one or two but usually it is within seven. As mentioned previously, choosing too many remedies can sometimes cloud the picture, which shouldn't have adverse effects on the remedy, but we may find it difficult to establish which remedies are working well. After the first course of treatment, which will last about two or three weeks, we may want to change the remedies we are using. If we are prescribing for others, this may be because after the second or third interview session we are beginning to identify hidden states of mind that were not apparent at first. Also, sometimes the healing process is like stripping away the mental layers of negative thought patterns, and when the remedies work to reveal another layer, this may indicate a change of remedy. This can be a positive sign that the healing process is gaining momentum and progressing well. Generally, the type remedy usually stays the same throughout the course of treatment, because this is based on the core personality that the person was born with, although it may not be apparent or dominant until adulthood.

It doesn't matter if we cannot spot an obvious type remedy. Sometimes the main personality trait may be more general and perhaps two or three type remedies are indicated, and these can change in dominance according to whatever people are experiencing in their lives at the time. For example, we all react differently to good and bad events and our personality can change accordingly. Personalities can also change dramatically over time. A quiet and introverted boy can turn into an angry and overly dominating adult and then into a loving and peaceful elderly man. We all have the capacity to change; impermanence is in the nature of all things. Again, we can use the flexibility of the remedies to counteract these changes by adapting our prescriptions accordingly.

Treatment Basics

Pure, still (not carbonated) mineral water seems to work best as a carrier of the healing life force. If mineral water isn't available, filtered water or water that has been boiled and cooled will work well. Normal tap water can also be used. Fruit juice, tea, coffee, and other drinks can also be carriers and are a good way of giving them to others, especially if they have not actually asked for the remedies but we feel they will help. (Obviously this is an area for debate, so decide for yourself if this is ethical or not.)

The remedies can be taken directly on the tongue from the stock bottle, but try not to touch the tongue with the dropper for obvious hygienic reasons.

If many remedies are indicated for a treatment, perhaps eight or nine, then we can either choose those that are most important and relevant at present, or use them all at once to provide a complete healing picture. If we choose the latter method, we can remove the less important remedies (i.e., those for the less dominant states of mind) from the combination as healing takes place and they are no longer required. We can also add new remedies each time we prepare a new treatment bottle as the healing process sometimes manifests states of mind that were not obvious at first. It is worth remembering that two or three remedies that go right to the heart of the matter can sometimes be more effective than eight or nine that skirt around the real issue, so accurate diagnosis and confidence in the choices is the key.

Using the Remedies — Short-term

When we have bought the remedies, it is very simple to prepare and administer them. If we want to treat a short-term illness, like a cold or a headache, or a temporary negative or unhappy state of mind, put two drops of the appropriate remedy into a small glass of still, pure mineral water, and sip it at intervals until the symptoms improve. Try to hold the water in the mouth for ten seconds or longer before swallowing. With experience we will know what works best for us. Sometimes it is best to finish the glass within fifteen to twenty minutes and sometimes it should last a few hours. We can also keep the glass by our bedside and sip it during the night if we wake up. Again, we can combine a few remedies into one glass. The remedies can also be taken directly on the tongue, straight from the stock bottle.

The typical dosage is two drops of each remedy in water taken three or four times a day, using more or less depending on how the symptoms respond. There is no limit to the amount used or frequency as there is no danger of side effects. You can make one glass last all day if that works best for you.

These two methods of using the remedies are ideal for short-term treatment. For example, we may wake up one morning and feel that we cannot face the day ahead. The thought of going to work makes us feel weak and depressed, a sort of Monday-morning sickness. Taking a couple of drops of Hornbeam would help energize us and make us feel more enthusiastic. If we are having problems waking and still feel drowsy after getting up, taking Clematis can help. If, when we get to work, someone is really irritating us, we could use Impatiens. Using the remedies in this way helps us deal with the changing moods, thoughts, and feelings of everyday life.

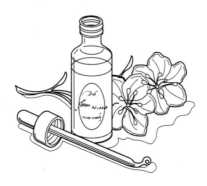

Example of a remedy stock bottle with dropper

If we have a short-term illness, a minor injury, or some sort of temporary emotional upset or worry, such as general depression or shock, we can choose remedies to relieve our symptoms and promote the healing process. Again, try to establish the predominant states of mind that accompany the illness or injury and choose the appropriate remedy. For example, someone with a cold might feel lethargic and apathetic. He or she might also feel despondent and want to be alone yet feel lonely. These "symptoms" would indicate Wild Rose, Gentian, and Water Violet. Someone else with the same cold virus might be pushing and straining to carry on, feeling vulnerable and weak. These symptoms would indicate Vervain and Centaury.

Both of these people need different remedies to get the best healing results, even though they have the same illness. If these states of mind are brought on only during illness, then using the right remedies can produce a swift recovery.

One of the great advantages of the Bach remedies over conventional medicine is that instead of concentrating on physical symptoms, healing takes place by helping the patient mentally and emotionally. These changes in attitude are the first sign that healing has begun. This also has a positive effect on those closest to the patient, such as family, friends, and caregivers, who are often under more stress if the patient is easily irritated or depressed.

Using the Remedies — Long-term

If we want to treat more long-term mental or physical conditions, it is not practical and even wasteful to use the same methods for more temporary conditions, as we can quickly use up whole bottles of each remedy. Instead, we need to make our own remedy bottle.

First, we need to buy one or two 30-milliliter dropper bottles, which can usually be obtained from a drug store, health food store, or herbalist supplier. Make sure the bottle is clean by filling it once or twice with hot, boiled water, and then rinsing with mineral water. Put two drops of each remedy indicated into the empty dropper bottle and fill it with still mineral water.

In this form, the minimum dosage is four drops on the tongue, four times a day. Hold the remedy on the tongue for a short time before swallowing. Again, do not touch the tongue with the dropper. This bottle should last about two to three weeks.

Once you have prepared the remedy, it is best to store it in a cool place, such as a refrigerator, and out of direct sunlight. When the bottle is empty, sterilize it, and rinse it out once or twice with spring water before reusing.

This was the method Dr. Bach recommended, and it is definitely the best way to treat any condition that lasts longer than a few days. We can take more than four drops four times a day if we need to. If we plan on taking a higher daily dose, we could prepare two treatment bottles at once and keep the one we are not using in the refrigerator until we need it.

A teaspoon of brandy can be added to the remedy bottle to keep it fresh. This is especially useful if it is not practical to keep the bottle in a refrigerator, or if tap water is used instead of mineral or spring water, which tends to stay fresh longer, up to two or three weeks. If you have access to a pure and clean supply of fresh spring water, this would be ideal for making your remedies, especially if the spring was once renown for its healing qualities.

If you do use brandy and are preparing the remedies for others, it is important to be aware that some people may be sensitive to alcohol or may not be able to take it for other reasons. The remedy stock bottles available over the counter do contain mainly brandy for preservative reasons; only a few drops of the original "mother tincture" (the main source of the healing energy held within each remedy) being required because of its potency. To avoid this, you will have to make the actual remedy yourself, preparing it from the appropriate plant. This is a wonderful thing to do if you have the time and access to the right plants and trees. (The exact methods and plants are explained in *The Bach Flower Remedies: Illustrations and Preparations*, published by C. W. Daniel Co. Ltd.)

Using the method of four drops, four times a day (at least), consistently floods the body and mind with the appropriate healing life force energy. The effectiveness of this constant supply of healing energy gains momentum the longer and more consistently we take the remedies. Over a few weeks we can see remarkable results.

Sometimes it may take longer, perhaps six weeks to two months, especially if the illness has been a long one. If we persist with the treatment, there can be a sudden improvement, even after several weeks of apparently little change. Perhaps this is because the healing energy needs time to build up in the system before it reaches a level that tips the balance toward good health.

Another way of taking the remedies is to buy a bottle of spring water (some people prefer glass, but plastic is okay), empty the contents into a sterile glass container, then put eight to ten drops of each of the chosen remedies into the treatment bottle, and refill with the spring water. Again, keep this bottle in the refrigerator or some other cool place out of direct sunlight. Sip a small glassful (4–8 fluid ounces) of this water four times a day, more if required, remembering to hold the remedy on the tongue for a while before swallowing.

We can take the remedies on a regular, long-term basis without using a dropper bottle. Simply put two drops of the chosen remedies into a glass of water and sip at intervals throughout the day. This can last all day with a fresh one made every morning. The obvious advantage to this is that we can vary the combination of remedies according to our daily needs. The remedy can also be taken in the middle of the night if we wake up. This is a good time to take it as our body and mind is more relaxed and open to receiving the healing energy. If we wake up after a bad dream we can use the appropriate remedy for fear (Mimulus, Rock Rose), shock (Star of Bethlehem), or loneliness (Water Violet,

Heather). Used in this way the remedies can be a great help to children if they are prone to bad dreams.

Once physical and mental equilibrium and good health are restored and well established, our own natural healing abilities return. We do not have to keep taking the remedies to maintain health unlike many conventional medicines. Occasionally, someone might need one or two more courses of treatment after an initial period of good health, which generally results in successful and permanent relief.

Making the Most of the Remedies

Remembering to take our remedies four times or more each day can be difficult. It is helpful to take it upon waking, at lunch, dinner, and just before going to bed. If you can spare the time, sitting quietly or lying down for a few minutes after taking the remedy can help, letting its healing energy enter your system. Try to relax and mentally connect and open up to the healing energy. It may actually feel like a spiral of energy coming from above or as a cushion of energy around the body. This sensation may wear off after a few minutes or it may stay for some time. The longer we take the remedies, the more we may become aware of this healing energy around us. We may feel our mind become clearer and feel more relaxed, less stressed, and more energized.

Sometimes after a few days treatment, some people may experience an emotional release connected with the healing process. This might be the result of a suppressed emotional response from years ago, a recent shock or accident, or it might be the release of accumulated stress gathered over the course of a long illness or a long period of difficult life experiences. This is a good sign that the remedies are doing their job and helping us work toward inner and outer health. This release may also take the form of laughing or any other emotional expression. Obviously this can have an effect on those around us, so if we are beginning to find our "voice" for the first time, and we want to express strong emotions like anger or love, we have to be careful and wise in our actions. Often these strong emotions, if they arise at all, are only passing phases, and it is often advisable to just to watch and allow them to "come through," remembering that they will simply pass in time.

When taking our remedies, we can think positive thoughts and affirmations such as "Every day I am becoming more whole, happy, and healthy." Or we could say a short prayer and ask for healing blessings. We could do a short visualization, imagining a spiral of pure healing energy entering our body and mind and renewing our health and vitality. We could see this energy as white, gold, deep blue, emerald green, or any other color that we feel is healing for us. We could visualize ourselves as relaxed, peaceful, healthy, deeply happy, and positive. Simple, childlike faith is the key to successful visualization. Remember when we were children and we imagined being someone else, maybe a doctor, athlete, or race car driver. When we played these roles we had light, happy mind; we really believed we were these people. This is a powerful way to use our mind to encourage good health and a positive outlook. Simply visualize the person we would like to be; enjoy and believe we are that person. Since our mind works through familiarity, the more we do this, the more it will become reality.

These methods may not be suitable for everyone so we have to use our own judgment and experience to know when to use them or recommend them to others. We also have to be practical and work within our limitations. There is no point visualizing climbing a mountain if we are severely disabled, unless this makes us feel good in some way. Our mind can also get bored with the same visualization, especially if we have to do it for a few weeks. For visualizations and affirmations to be effective, they have to be of great interest and relevance to the individual. They have to be creative and evolve and change with the healing process.

Exceptions to this are the healing mantras and meditations used in Buddhism. They seem to have a special effect on the mind that naturally holds and increases our interest. The more they are practiced, the more they take us deeper into our own nature and give us the power to deal directly with those issues that are the source of our problems. (Mantra meditations are discussed in chapter 10.)

It is worth remembering that Dr. Bach had great faith in the remedies. He believed that if the patient truly and deeply wanted to be well, the remedies would bring this about. This confidence in the power of the remedies is very important if we are prescribing for others. The remedies can have great power on their own, but if we can support and encourage the patient's confidence in the remedies through our own belief in their healing power, then this can really make a positive difference.

Dr. Bach found that the patients who made the greatest effort on their own stood the best chances of recovery. So if we can encourage people not to worry and to be positive and to help themselves in whatever way they can, then this can add momentum to the healing process.

Using the Remedies Externally

Remedies can be used directly on the skin as well as on the tongue. Crab Apple is good for skin problems when they are accompanied by feelings of being dirty or unclean. Skin irritation can be treated with Impatiens, if the mental state is frustration and impatience. Other remedies can be used in the same way.

To use externally, put two to four drops of the remedy into a glass of water, and apply this directly to the area or with a cloth. The remedy could also be applied as a salve by using an appropriate holding cream, such as a hand cream or moisturizer (nothing overly scented). The remedy could also be placed in the water we wash in (four drops) or take a bath in (eight to ten drops). This might be especially useful if someone is experiencing nervous tremors and the predominant mindset indicates

Aspen (for general fear or worry) and Scleranthus (for indecision and unsteadiness). If someone has strained a muscle or twisted an ankle and the dominant state of mind indicates Vervain (for mental strain), we could prepare a compress and apply it to the strained area as well as giving the remedy orally. Sometimes Rock Water or Impatiens can also be relevant for such cases.

Rescue Remedy

The Rescue Remedy was devised by Dr. Bach to be used mainly in emergency situations or after an accident, physical injury, or shock. Many people carry a bottle of this wherever they go, and it has been an invaluable life-saver in countless instances. The Rescue Remedy is made up of five of the Bach remedies: Clematis for faintness, drowsiness, and sleepiness; Star of Bethlehem for shock; Rock Rose for extreme fear or terror; Impatiens for irritation and frustration; and Cherry Plum for extreme mental pressure. This is a wonderful remedy to use in any emergency or in any daily situation where we are worried, irritated, drowsy, frightened, shocked, or under a lot of pressure. For example, we could use it before and after an exam, interview, a confrontational situation, or giving a public speech.

Rescue Remedy is available just like the other remedies. To use, simply put four drops directly on the tongue or in a glass of water. It can also be dropped directly onto the skin for minor cuts, burns, and insect bites and stings. There is also a Rescue Remedy cream available, which is very useful as well.

Treating Children

Generally, we treat children in the same way we treat adults, simply by prescribing according to their mental and emotional state. Children often respond very positively to the remedies, and healing can often be swifter than adults. Consequently, we may need to change the remedy combination more quickly than normal. The obvious difference in treating young children and animals is that they cannot easily express their feelings clearly. However, mood is often displayed through behavior. Common emotions like anger, fear, and shyness can be easily recognized just by watching how children play, how they react to meeting people, and how they behave when they are unhappy. Like all people, when children and animals are ill, their common states of mind may give way to unusual ones, and we can prescribe the remedies according to those states of mind that are most obvious. For example, a quiet and lonely child would need Water Violet, a sleepy child would suit Clematis, a shy child Mimulus, a domineering child Vine, and a demanding child Chicory.

Children's personalities can change a lot. There are plenty of challenging experiences throughout childhood and adolescence, so if we are a parent and we want to help our children by using the remedies, our first priority is to keep the lines of communication open with our children. If we cannot understand and except them for who they are and allow them to grow as nature intended, they will naturally turn away from us and we will be unable to help them. However, if they grow in a loving, encouraging, and supportive environment where the parents are open, loving, and communicative to each other and to their children, then there is hope for the children to become similarly well-adjusted adults.

Children can be prone to all sorts of extreme emotions. Many remedies can be helpful such as Holly for envy or jealousy, Willow for sulking, or Vervain and Impatiens for strain and frustration. Gentian is useful for those who give up easily, Wild Rose for the apathetic and lazy, and Walnut to help with the rapid changes that many children face while growing up.

The remedies can be added to their milk or formula, if they are still on the bottle, or treated directly from the stock bottle, although some children might not like the taste. They can also be added to fruit juice or other types of drink children prefer.

The Bach Rescue Remedy is also helpful to have around with children. It can be useful for any kind of minor physical injury such as falls, cuts, and bruises, and any sort of mental and emotional upset. It can quickly calm fears and shocks and generally help soothe upset children—including their wound-up parents.

Treating Plants

Plants can also be successfully treated by placing a few drops of the right remedy in their water before watering. Crab apple is good for disease, Willow for a plant that looks droopy, and Gentian for a plant that continually gets better and then worse. Gorse is for one that has given up completely, Olive for those that lack vitality, Oak for those that struggle on, and Star of Bethlehem for bushes and trees that have been excessively pruned. These are just general rules, so use whichever remedy you feel is appropriate. If you are unsure, try the Rescue Remedy.

Seven

Bach Remedies for Animals

This chapter begins with an article by Dr. Anna Maria Scholey. She is a holistic veterinarian who uses flower essences to treat animals. It is followed by several stories from Bach flower practitioners and animal lovers who have had positive experiences with the remedies on their own animals.

Advice from a Holistic Veterinarian

Dr. Edward Bach believed that diseases of the body come about as a result of imbalances or negativity at the level of the soul. By correcting that problem, healing would result and the patient would heal on all levels. The flower remedies act to balance the emotional and spiritual body, and cause a gentle healing by bringing the body back in balance with itself. They act almost as healing catalysts. Animals respond just as well to the Bach Flower Remedies as people do, and they seem to have similar emotional imbalances that can be corrected with the appropriate remedy.

By becoming familiar with the thirty-eight flower essences, you can treat almost every condition with these alone. Each essence treats a particular imbalance and they can be used alone or in combination, depending what the problem is. It is often more effective to use a single essence, as this is more focused. It is possible to use more, but the maximum recommended number of remedies to combine is seven, and it is best to use as few as possible for maximum results.

One well-chosen flower remedy will be more powerful in its action than several less well-selected ones. In practice, three or four related remedies seem to work well together and a combination might be made up. For example, treating fear needs the following three Bach Flower Remedies: Mimulus for fear of known causes, Aspen for groundless fears, and Rock Rose for acute fear or panic. Together these three will cover most aspects of fear. If the fear was due to some trauma in the past, then Star of Bethlehem may be added, as this helps release any shock and trauma from the body, however long ago it took place.

The remedies can be given by adding two drops of each remedy that is indicated into a one-ounce dropper bottle, fill with spring water, and add a dropper or two of a preservative such as brandy or apple cider vinegar. When a remedy is made for people, alcohol is used as a preservative, but I find that for small animals, like rabbits, it is best to use plain spring water. Four drops of this mixture can then be given on the gums four times a day, for about six to eight weeks, to achieve the desired effect.

The most useful Bach remedy of all is Rescue Remedy, which is actually a combination of five other remedies. They act synergistically to calm stress and fear and treat shock or trauma. It is an invaluable addition to the first aid kit that any pet owner would find useful. It can be used before visiting the vet office or after any kind of injury. It will often revive animals that are in shock and maintain them on their way to the vet and help them recover. It is obviously not a replacement for immediate veterinary care. It has definitely saved many animals and is totally safe. It can even be sprayed onto the skin or ears with a spray bottle, and it will still have a beneficial effect. For animals that are unconscious, the safest way is to put a little of the remedy onto the ear or just one or two drops onto the gums, being careful not to let any go down the throat. Rescue Remedy also helps animals recover from anesthesia and surgery.

There are five essences in the Rescue Remedy: Star of Bethlehem for trauma and numbness; Clematis to prevent passing out; Rock Rose for panic; Impatiens for tension and irritability; and Cherry Plum to prevent feelings of losing control.

To prepare the Rescue Remedy, add four drops to a one-ounce glass dropper bottle filled with spring water, and shake. It is best to make this immediately before use as the mixture will not keep long. Three or four drops of this mixture can be given orally or placed on the gums every five minutes until a response is seen. Rescue Remedy can also be mixed with the animal's drinking water during any time of stress. In this case, it is best to add ten drops every time the water is changed.

Emotions and Behavior

As described above, flower remedies and essences have many varied uses, but they act mainly on the higher emotional levels. The body is affected very much by the emotions and the mind, and by healing at a deeper level, flower remedies can shift illnesses, either alone or more often in combination with other forms of treatment. For example, skin problems may manifest in animals during times of anxiety and stress, such as when a new pet or a new baby enters the household. The physical symptoms may be due to jealousy, anger, resentment, loneliness, or other emotions, but by careful questioning, an idea of what may be going on can be determined and a remedy mixture made up to address the root cause of the problem. In the meantime, the skin may also need to be treated, but by addressing the issue at both of these levels, the end results are much better than merely treating the skin alone.

Flower remedies can help with behavioral problems, such as biting and aggression. It is important to combine the remedy with training and behavior modification. Both of these approaches are enhanced by the flower remedies. Fear, such as a fear of thunderstorms or a general lack of confidence, is a common problem in animals, and can also be calmed by suitable remedies. Animals that have been rescued or abused in the past often benefit from the use of appropriate flower essences, as they can help to restore confidence and build trust.

Rescue Remedy, combined with the remedy Aconite, makes a wonderful calming essence that can be used on wild animals and for animal rehabilitation. As mentioned before, it works well on any kind of stress or fear and definitely helps with the survival rate in these situations. A few drops of the combined Rescue Remedy and Aconite on the gums, or even on or behind the ear of the rescued animal, will calm them down and make them easier to handle. A dropper of the combination can be put into the daily water for rescued animals to help them withstand the stress of captivity and make them more manageable. The combination can be similarly used for more domesticated animals.

Other problems such as pets that tend to wander away from home, cats that urinate and defecate all over the house, or animals that suffer from separation anxiety can all benefit from the flower remedies. Often for the improvement to be permanent, though, other changes have to be made. Some problems are related to other animals in the household (territorial behavior), and this may persist as long as the other animal is present. Nevertheless, appropriate flower essences can help alleviate and resolve many of these situations, again combined most effectively with behavior modification and possible changes to the living environment.

Remedies for Specific Situations

Here is a list of some of the Bach flower essences and their indications for animals, along with some essences from other companies. (Bach = Bach Flower Remedies; FES = Flower Essence Society*)

Aspen

This remedy is for animals that are very fearful for no apparent reason, and who are very sensitive to anxiety and apprehension. They may tremble with fear and anxiety without any obvious causation. (Bach)

Bleeding Heart

This is for grieving animals that have suffered a loss of either another animal or person. It also helps animals

---

* Dr. Scholey recommends some remedies that are not in the Bach repertory. These are detailed on the Flower Essence Societies website. Visit the author's website for the link. FES is a general body for people interested in flower remedies.

who have never recovered from a loss or grief that happened in the past. (FES)

Centaury

Centaury is for animals that are overly submissive and eager to please, tending to be bullied by other animals. It is also for animals that grovel and urinate from submissive behavior when petted. (Bach)

Chamomile

This is a calming remedy that helps fractious and irritable animals. It is especially useful if they are teething and for calming terrible temper tantrums. (FES)

Cherry Plum

This remedy is for animals that cannot control their behavior, such as aggression and biting, who tend to have violent impulses toward other animals and people, and are even dangerous. (Bach)

Chicory

Chicory is for the overly possessive and maternal animal that wants attention all the time and is also jealous of other animals or people who might compete with them for affection. (Bach)

Crab Apple

This is for cleansing the body and getting rid of toxins. This remedy acts on the physical body more than any of the other essences and is good for any situation where cleansing is required. (Bach)

Gentian

Gentian is for animals that are easily discouraged and give up easily. For example, in training programs, they give up if they make even a small mistake. (Bach)

Heather

This remedy is for animals that hate to be left alone, who suffer from separation anxiety. These animals tend to be quite vocal and may whine and cry a lot if left alone. (Bach)

Impatiens

This is for the impatient, fast moving, hyperactive animal that never seems to slow down. These animals can be snappy and irritable, and they tend to rush ahead or pull on the leash. (Bach)

Larch

Larch is for animals that lack self-confidence and tend to be timid and shy. It can help animals that need to perform in the show ring but don't have the confidence to show themselves well. (Bach)

Mimulus

This remedy is for animals that are scared of known things, such as thunderstorms or other animals or people. It helps them overcome their fears and be less timid and scared of the world. (Bach)

Olive

Olive is for animals that are exhausted and drained by a long strain or a difficult illness, such as a chronic disease. This will help them handle the ordeal better and become stronger again. (Bach)

Pink Yarrow

This helps protect animals from negative emotional energy, such as that during a divorce, stressful family situations, or when another animal or person is sick or draining their energy reserves. (FES)

Rescue Remedy

This is the single most useful flower remedy combination. It helps with any kind of stress or trauma, such as accidents, birthing, illness, stress, and recovery after a seizure. (Bach)

Rock Rose

This is useful for animals that are very scared and prone to panic attacks for no known reason. They become totally rigid with fear and tend to be highly strung and nervous. (Bach)

Self Heal

This is a wonderful remedy by itself or in combination with other essences. It helps stimulate the innate healing reserves of the body and improves health during any illness. (FES)

Special Yarrow Formula

This formula helps protect animals and people from negative external influences, such as environmental pollution, toxins, electromagnetic energy, and other factors. (FES)

Star of Bethlehem

This remedy is for animals that have suffered any kind of trauma, emotional or physical, such as an accident or abuse. It helps them recover from this shock, however long ago it took place. (Bach)

Tiger Lily

This remedy helps with aggression and animals that tend to bite and snap. It helps them be less hostile and opens them up to learning to cooperate with others. (FES)

Vervain

This is good for the overly enthusiastic animal that is overbearing and high strung. It helps calm hyperactivity and restlessness and is for the animal that wears people out by their excess energy. (Bach)

Vine

This remedy helps with the dominant animal who wants to be the boss of all the other animals and people. They are bullies to other animals around them and hate to be disciplined. (Bach)

Walnut

This is an extremely useful remedy for any time of transition, such as moving house, becoming pregnant, adjusting to new animals or family members, or going to a new situation. (Bach)

Water Violet

This remedy tends to suit cats that are unusually introverted and detached, and it helps open them up to be more friendly and outgoing and less aloof and emotionally distant. (Bach)

Wild Oat

This helps the restless animal that never seems to know what they want or settles down into anything. It helps them focus their energies and be less scattered in their approach to life. (Bach)

Willow

This remedy helps with resentment and bitterness, and often helps cats that urinate everywhere due to a change in the household, such as the arrival of another animal or a baby.

—*Dr. Anna Maria Scholey*

Confident Cats

When we were temporarily living in a rented house my two female cats were savagely attacked by a very large, territorially minded male cat. For four to five months they were both too terrified to go outside, preferring the safety of using an indoor litter box to venturing out into the garden. Instead of two normally active cats I had two couch potatoes.

By a stroke of bad luck, when we moved into our new house, their first trip into the garden coincided with a visit from our new neighbor's cat who, although a peaceful animal, looked just like the one that attacked them. One glance and they both shot back indoors, refusing all my blandishments to get them to even look out through the cat door.

I puzzled for a time over how to help them. As cats do not drink and both of mine are very hostile to taking drops, I first diluted some Rescue Remedy and saturated two pieces of their favorite food (raw rabbit) with it, and gave each one a piece four times a day. The braver cat was out and about in the garden by the following morning and presented no further problems. Her more timid sister would look outside but nothing more, so I made up a remedy using Mimulus, Larch, and Star of Bethlehem. She appeared calmer and sat on the window sill, observing the garden with keen interest, so I continued on with Chestnut Bud and Honeysuckle. After two doses, the "cure" was complete, and she was out in the garden with her sister, establishing her own claim to the new territory.

—Valerie Walker-Dendle
Bach flower practioner, counselor/therapist

Dog Story

This is a brief story of our dog Bilbo's miraculous recovery while on holiday in southern Ireland. On Friday afternoon, he became ill for no known reason except that he had a history of stomach problems, so it could have been something he had eaten. Looking back, he had been a little quiet all day. His stomach then went into a spasm and stayed that way until halfway through the night.

Obviously in pain, he could not find anywhere comfortable to rest. He vomited his breakfast, undigested, and was sick once or twice more. I decided to stay up with him. Luckily he wanted to drink, so each time he drank a little water I put in four drops of Rescue Remedy. I also gave him healing (as Dr. Bach himself did on many occasions) throughout the night. I vividly remember the point when the spasms in his stomach and legs stopped. After a little while he slept.

We were due to return home the next morning. He just layed flat during the ferry ride and wasn't doing so well. Halfway through the three and a half-hour journey home in the car, he seemed to recover some strength, and by the time we got home, he jumped out of the car and did a tour of the garden, announcing to all that he was back. By Tuesday he made a full and quite miraculous recovery. Both my husband and I were surprised at the speed of his full recovery.

—*Sheila Bennett*

Healing Two Dogs with One Bowl

I use the remedies as part of my everyday life. I have used them with my goldfish, plants, children, and especially, my dogs. One of my dogs, a twelve-year-old English springer spaniel, suddenly became aggressive and would not let my other dog, a thirteen-year-old Weimaraner, in the same room as him. He generally became unfriendly with all of us. I had discovered the previous weekend that he had become completely deaf and took this to be the problem. I made him a Bach remedy treatment bottle, which I began putting in his water and food. It consisted of Vine (his type remedy), Aspen, Rock Rose, and Walnut. I thought these would be appropriate for what he was experiencing.

He changed almost immediately, back to his loveable self. Obviously his hearing has not been restored, but he seems to be coping with his problem now. There has also been a positive side effect of this treatment. Our Weimaraner is very shaky on his back legs at times. If he goes up the stairs, he is too afraid to come down as he has fallen down them a few times and so then has to be carried. Since I put the remedies into the water bowl that they both drink from, he came up the stairs the other night and walked down them with no problems. I can only assume that the Rock Rose (for terror) worked for him as well.

—*Teresa Munro*

Eight

38 Bach Flower Remedies

As Dr. Bach taught, the easiest way to recognize the remedies that are relevant and accurate for an individual is to assess which negative states of mind predominate—not the positive states of mind that need to be encouraged. If we tried to prescribe in the latter way, it would take much longer and we would probably not be so accurate. It is generally much easier to spot a negative state of mind than a positive one, mainly because when things are going well we tend not to analyze ourselves, we just carry on as normal and enjoy our life. It is only when things go wrong and we are unhappy that we stop and look more closely at ourselves and our life and ask questions: "Why do I feel like this?" "Why have things gone wrong? "What can I do about this?" It is easier to spot negative minds in others because they are more obvious than positive ones. We have a whole range of expressions and vocabulary to cover the negative emotions and thoughts, but when we are positive, all we generally show is a smile and all we can say is that we are happy

We also probably have a natural ability to spot any kind of negative emotion quickly. Perhaps this is part of our natural makeup. One of the basic human functions is to survive by spotting any kind of mental, emotional, or physical danger quick enough so that we can act to protect ourselves. Evolution works on the survival of the fittest, and since human beings have always been sociable creatures, learning to spot what was going on within the minds of others was a necessary part of self-preservation and success within the family group or clan. The earliest humans had to learn to communicate to survive; living in sociable groups was far safer than living alone, and there was more chance of regular food. So again, we had to learn to recognize others emotions and thought patterns to survive, especially those that were negative like fear, anger, or suspicion.

We also seem to find negative minds more interesting than positive ones. Look at the type of things people watch on television. For example, if soap operas only had positive people leading happy lives, would anybody watch them? Actually, we can use programs like soap operas to help us practice identifying type remedies as they so often have clearly defined characters that have obvious leanings toward certain remedies. The dominating type might be Vine, the weak type Centaury, the shy type Mimulus, those who are always asking others advice Cerato, those who hide their worries behind a smile Agrimony, and those who keep repeating the same mistakes Chestnut Bud. We can also try to spot which remedies are relevant for the changing mental states that people show, i.e., irritation, anger, jealousy, overconcern for others, depression, terror, guilt, or loneliness. All these are classic indications of specific remedies.

Motivation and Dedication

There are two simple things practiced in Buddhist healing that we can do to make our healing actions more powerful and meaningful. If we are planning to make a remedy for ourselves or others we can begin with a short prayer, affirmation, or mental intention, and finish with a brief "dedication."

Intention is everything. Our intention, or motivation, is what creates our karma. As mentioned before, everything we do, say, and think, every action of body, speech, and mind creates a potential in the mind for a corresponding physical, verbal, or mental reaction in the future. It also creates the habit or tendency for us to repeat such actions and an increased wish or compulsion to keep performing similar negative actions. If we perform negative actions, we can expect negative reactions sooner or later. Also, if we generally have a negative approach to life, we are more likely to create the conditions that attract problems and difficult circumstances. Likewise, the positive energy we create by developing patience and kindness, or preparing a Bach remedy for someone, will return to us as a positive experience in one form or another.

If we set a positive mental intention before we perform any type of healing action, including making a remedy, this will increase the power of our good karma. If this intention is wise and heartfelt, the consequences of our actions can benefit countless living beings, even though we cannot directly see this.

Basically if our motivation is to benefit others rather than ourselves, this will create powerful and positive karma.

To set an intention, we just need to sit quietly for a few minutes, calm the mind, and think of those people we would like to benefit. Then we can simply think or pray the following passages:

> *Through the force of these healing actions may*
> *(name the people you are thinking of) find lasting*
> *happiness and good health.*

Or even more powerfully:

> *May every living being benefit from these healing*
> *actions for their greatest good.*

Once we have finished preparing the remedy, we can dedicate our positive actions or good karma. Dedication is similar to intention. If we consciously dedicate or direct this positive energy for a specific purpose, this can be a powerful way of manifesting our intentions, achieving our goals, and accelerating our spiritual or personal growth. Whenever we create positive energy or good karma by helping others, or by consciously developing positive states of mind, we can dedicate this energy.

Choosing a purpose or direction for a dedication is similar to creating an intention. If we can choose a purpose that will benefit many people, then this wish will be fulfilled more easily than a purely selfish purpose. To dedicate after any positive action, we can simply think or pray the following:

> *May this positive energy be fully dedicated for the greatest good of all living beings.*

Or:

> *May every living being benefit from this positive energy.*

Perhaps the greatest goals we could wish for are the following:

> *Through the force of this positive energy may every living being be released from suffering and may we all find true lasting happiness swiftly and easily.*

And/or:

*Through the force of these positive actions may my
wisdom and compassion continually increase for
the benefit of others.*

Dedicating the positive energy created by our
actions only takes a short time, but this small gesture is
a very special practice. Another idea is that if we have
many remedies to prepare or a day of healing ahead of
us, we can set our intention in the morning and dedicate in the evening.

We can easily waste or destroy the potential of positive actions, or good karma, simply by developing negative states of mind like anger, guilt, or jealousy. Sincere
and heartfelt dedication is like "banking" or protecting
the potential of our positive actions for our own and
others' benefit. In this way, the potential of our good
thoughts, words, and deeds can only increase and will
produce excellent results for everyone in the future.

This rest of this chapter details each of the thirty-
eight remedies, beginning with a brief "key word"
description to help point healers in the right direction.
Then there is a more detailed analysis giving the main
mental and emotional symptoms that are relevant to
each remedy as well as the positive aspects (remedy
effects) that will arise through successful treatment.

Agrimony

Agrimonia eupatoria
Hidden worries; outwardly cheerful

Agrimony types hide their problems behind humor or faked cheerfulness. They find it difficult to talk openly about their problems, preferring to keep things bottled up inside. They often feel most at peace or "themselves" when they are alone or with those they really trust, when they can let the mask of cheerfulness drop and finally express what is on their mind. It can take a long time for the Agrimony type to accept and trust another person. He or she tends to keep people at arm's length emotionally.

They find it difficult to deal with other people's problems, especially if they are deep emotional ones. They may try to change the subject if they feel uncomfortable and try to pass things off lightly, saying things like, "Don't worry, I'm sure everything will be okay," or "Well that's life." For them, this is a way of avoiding their own inner worries and the prospect of having to face them or talk openly about them. They are often afraid of showing deep emotion in front of others and will present the "stiff upper lip" in any stressful situation rather than cry, get angry, or be openly loving. However, they do not have any problem laughing in public, although genuine laughter can often lead to tears if they are with a trusted friend, as their mask slips and their true emotions surface.

Agrimony types are often the joker, the person who always seems to be in a good mood. They usually appear cheerful, bubbly, and friendly, as if they do not have a care in the world. If they are asked how they are, they will often reply with a light breezy remark like, "Oh, fine." If asked about a specific problem or crisis they are having, they will give a brief answer and gloss over any deeper worries with a self-deprecating joke and nervous or false laughter. Then they may change the subject quickly so that they feel more comfortable. Consequently, they can be quite nervous, tense, and jittery people, finding it difficult to genuinely relax in the presence of new company. It usually takes them some time to trust and feel safe with new friends.

They are most relaxed and at peace with themselves when with close family or friends. Some Agrimony types can only be that comfortable when they are alone. Extreme types can convince themselves that nothing is wrong to the extent that they bury emotional problems deep within. Eventually, these may surface as a physical or mental illness, sometimes depression or a nervous or emotional breakdown. They may often use distractions like working hard to help them ignore their inner problems. They are also prone to addictions like drugs, alcohol, food, and destructive relationships—anything to hide or dull the pain and unhappiness within. Being the center of attention by being amusing, attractive, and charming can be like a drug for them, helping them forget their inner difficulties and preventing conversation from moving to profound or emotionally deep subjects.

When that happens, they are uncomfortable and try to change the topic of conversation, crack a joke, become quiet, or leave to talk to someone else.

Often Agrimony symptoms may arise due to emotional trauma during childhood or adolescence. If at that time they did not know or were not taught how to deal with such problems in a healthy way, they may have simply coped by pushing down or burying their emotions. The longer these emotions are buried, the more frightening the prospect is of allowing them to come out. Generally speaking, if children see that this is how their parents deal with problems, then there is a good chance they will adopt these habits, too. They can even try to appear cheerful, putting on a brave face when dealing with extreme difficulties, illness, or loss. Trying to appear happy while inside they are in great misery makes things even worse and puts them under great strain.

Remedy Effects

Regular doses of Agrimony can help these people to be more relaxed, open, and honest. The mask begins to drop, and problems they are holding within gradually surface and dissipate, sometimes with a series of gentle emotional releases. They find it easier to talk openly and honestly about their problems, hopes, and wishes. Agrimony helps them to be more trusting of others and at peace with themselves, whether with company or alone. This is a wonderful remedy that many people can benefit from as we are all a little like this sometimes.

Aspen

Populus tremula

Nervous, vague, and nonspecific
worries or fears

The Aspen tree is sometimes called the "trembling tree," which is a good indication of the Aspen personality type. Aspen types can be quite nervous people. Due to their nervousness, they can appear to be quick, unsure, and shaky. They often lack self-confidence. In extreme cases, this nervousness can lead to exhaustion and subsequent illness. They have a general sense of worry. They may not necessarily be worried or frightened about something specific, just generally apprehensive. They can be superstitious and dwell on negative things. They think that bad things will come their way; nothing specifically bad, just generally that being alive is worrisome and the future foreboding.

They may say things like, "Things don't look good," "I think something bad might happen," or "I have a bad feeling about this." Mainly they are worriers for no good reason. Often, the worst time for them is that leading up to a stressful event that they cannot avoid, such as public speaking. It is the anticipation they hate—not knowing how things are going to turn out. This unsettles them and leaves them feeling frightened, vulnerable, and, sometimes, physically sick.

Sometimes Aspen types resort to smoking, drinking, or other sources of external "comfort" to help calm their nerves and get them through the day. Sometimes they cannot sleep as their worries and dread can increase at night. The dark is often associated with the unknown, and it is this aspect of fear that causes the most distress. Perhaps they are afraid of their own courage and what developing this quality might bring. They just want a quiet life in a small world that they can control and feel safe in.

In extreme cases, Aspen types may be overwhelmed by fear and dread that something terrible might happen. They can become on-edge, jumpy, and easily scared. Their minds can create all sorts of imaginary fears that change quickly, especially at night.

Remedy Effects

Aspen is one of the remedies for courage. Developing courage will break down the walls of fear and vulnerability and leads to a more open and confident approach to life. This remedy can help these people find inner strength and freedom from worry. They will be more able to face and enjoy life with a positive, strong, and relaxed attitude. This remedy can also be useful for children who may, for example, not want to go to bed, go to school, or meet new people. It is not because they are afraid of these actual events, but their anticipation and foreboding of what might happen that holds them back, seeking security in the arms of their parents.

Beech

Fagus sylvatica

Critical; lacking tolerance and empathy

These people do not suffer fools easily. Beech types often have high standards, and if others don't match up to these, they are often looked down upon for falling short of their expectations. Parents who are severe Beech types can be quite strict and can pass these traits onto their children. Children can often feel inadequate and unworthy if they feel they do not meet their parents' high standards.

They generally have a lack of empathy toward others and find it difficult to understand another person's point of view. They are often traditionalists and find it difficult to understand why anyone would want to live their life in an unusual way. Perhaps it threatens their sense of control; they feel more secure when things are "in place."

They can be well-organized people and want everything in place where it should be. They get annoyed if someone borrows something and doesn't put it back where it belongs. They have difficulty being spontaneous and creative. They like to run a tight ship and keep to routines and schedules.

Beech types are perfectionists and might say things like, "If a job's got to be done, it's got to be done right," "I wouldn't have done it like that," or "You should have done it like this." They can be quite unbending in their point of view, and the more people try to show them that they are wrong, the more adamant they are that they are right. They find it difficult to say they are sorry and admit that they might be wrong or that another point of view might be right. They might appear cold, distant, unloving, and lonely. They may have difficulty expressing affection and talking about their emotions. In fact, they tend to be more "head" than "heart" people. When a severe Beech type is hugged, he or she often tenses up or recoils.

Elderly people often show these qualities more obviously than younger people and, generally, men more than women. Beech types can appear to be patient and tolerant on the outside, while inside they have their own fixed principles and have no intention of changing. The classic extreme Beech types are often racist, sexist, ageist, and homophobic. Sometimes they can appear liberal, but when we get to know them better, we may find that they are very strict liberalists and can't understand anyone who isn't.

Remedy Effects

The Beech remedy helps these people become more open and tolerant and interested in others. It helps them develop empathy, understanding, and the wish to learn from others. The transformation in some people after taking this remedy is wonderful to see. They visibly become warmer, more communicative, and friendly people. Their ability to appreciate another point of view should increase and they should also become more supportive and encouraging of others' ideas and wishes.

Centaury

Centaurium umbellatum

Weak; easily influenced; overly willing servant

The Centaury person is generally not a leader; in fact, they are just the opposite. They like to be part of a team, following orders rather than giving them. They dislike responsibility and prefer to take a back seat, letting others make decisions for them to follow. They are often kind, gentle, and quiet people. They do not like to "rock the boat" or cause trouble for others in case they draw attention to themselves. They are willing helpers and certainly would never go out of their way to hurt others. If someone were to hurt them, they would accept it without wanting revenge or feeling anger. They are more likely to cry quietly than get angry.

Others often treat the extreme Centaury types badly; they get taken advantage of and used. They find it difficult to speak up and demand respect from others, so, consequently, others find it difficult to treat them with respect. They find it difficult to say no and usually say yes to any request for help or command, even if they really do not want to. This leaves them feeling even more weak and powerless, and some may develop a hatred of power or overt strength.

They can become exhausted by overwork. If they spend too much time in the presence of those who want to control them, they can easily lose what little self-worth they have and become a servant. In this way, they lose their own sense of self and finally only identify themselves as being a server. They lose their self-respect and other people look upon them as weak, pathetic, and ineffectual. Often what they say is ignored and, sometimes, even laughed at.

Centaury types also find it difficult to ask for help, even when they really need it. They do not like to be a nuisance to anyone. They would prefer to suffer than cause an inconvenience.

Remedy Effects

Centaury helps these people develop self-respect, strength, and independence. This remedy encourages a sense of self-worth and the ability to be firm and fair when the need arises. A good symbol for the positive qualities of this remedy is the lion: courage and strength tempered with the wisdom to know when to use them. The effects are often quite dramatic on people who react to illness in a weak and submissive way. It gives them a mental and emotional boost and restores their strength and will to get well. This is a real life-affirming remedy.

Cerato

Ceratostigma willmottiana

Indecision; asks the advice and opinions of others

Cerato is one of the remedies for indecision. Cerato types are unsure of themselves and find it difficult to have confidence in their own judgment. Therefore, they are easily influenced by others. One of the classic Cerato indications is a lack of confidence in their own abilities to make decisions. They find it difficult to be the leader and have far more confidence in the decision-making abilities of anyone but themselves.

They will tend to seek the advice of others rather than make up their own minds. They will often ask for suggestions and say things like, "What do you think I should do?" or "How would you deal with this problem?" This constant habit of seeking others for advice does not actually help them and, in fact, causes them more confusion. When they finally make a decision, they will continue to question it, often changing their minds several times before they finally decide one way or another. Even after a final decision is made and a course of action irreversible, they will continue to wonder how things might have been if they had done things differently. They will look to the opinions of others to help them, saying things like, "Do you think I did the right thing?" or "Do you think I should have done things differently?"

Cerato types often take the wrong path in life. Cerato children are easily swayed by their parents and often find themselves fulfilling the desires of others instead of answering their own true calling. This can cause them to be real fashion victims by always wearing or doing what the latest trends dictate. They also experience a lot of self-doubt and often extol the virtues of others who they would like to emulate, especially those who seem to know exactly what they are doing and where they are going.

A typical Cerato might show extreme symptoms when faced with major issues in life, like choosing a career, looking for a new place to live, or making relationship decisions. Because they feel so confused and unhappy when faced with taking a certain course of action, they will often put off the final decision as long as possible, leading to a quick judgment that is often done for them.

Remedy Effects

The Cerato remedy helps people become more clear, confident, and decisive. They will still seek the advice of others but in a positive way. Their minds are open to new ideas but not swayed just because another person's will is strong. They will know what is right for them and have the confidence in their own judgment to follow through with positive actions. This remedy helps people create clarity in the mind and confidence in decision making.

Cherry Plum

Prunus cerasifera

Fear of insanity, of the mind giving way

People suffering from the symptoms that suggest Cherry Plum are likely to be quite mentally or emotionally strained. They feel they cannot cope anymore and are frightened that they will go mad, or that their mind will be damaged in some way.

This remedy is also indicated when there is the impulse to do harm to oneself or to another. There is a definite lack of rationality. Cherry Plum types often feel commanded by their thoughts and impulses. There is often a fear of losing control that causes them great distress and a terrible feeling that they are going to "crack." These feelings are sometimes bottled up, and they are often frightened to talk about this for fear that others might think that they are losing their mind. This only makes things worse and puts more internal pressure on them.

Sometimes they may feel they are a burden to others who are worrying about them. Their wild, impulsive thoughts may turn to suicide as a way of relieving the mental distress. In mild states, they appear to be dreamy and not really "here." They are wrapped up in themselves as if in a world of their own. Consequently, they show little genuine interest in the problems of others, sometimes especially those closest to them.

The Cherry Plum condition can follow a long period of stress or any extremely traumatic experience or shock to the system. Sometimes it can run in families and not show itself until sometime during adulthood.

Remedy Effects

Many sufferers of mental illness can benefit from this remedy. It brings relief from the mental strain and fear of a nervous breakdown. It promotes a sense of inner strength, stability, peace, and mental well-being. There is often a great sense of relief on the faces of those who take Cherry Plum, accompanied by a renewed sense of hope and the feeling that they can go on. The remedy can also be useful for brief periods of a lack of mental control like angry outbursts, constant crying, or other strong, uncontrolled emotions. Cherry Plum is also for people who are prone to the fear of losing control when faced with a stressful situation.

Chestnut Bud

Æsculus hippocastanum

Always repeating the same mistake;
not learning from experience

Chestnut Bud is an ideal remedy for those who are trapped in a cycle of repetitive behavior. They find it hard to learn from experience, making the same mistakes many times before they finally realize that another course of action might be better. This can be quite a damaging state of mind, especially if it results in, for example, a series of damaging relationships, all with the same destructive qualities.

Sometimes these people do not realize that they are making the same mistakes. They can be quite naive and live in a semifantasy world where reality is not always welcome. They may tend to reject or avoid the advice of others, especially if it threatens their own views on life. Even if they are aware they are making the same mistakes, they cannot help themselves, even if they know that there is a strong chance that they will be hurt or that they will hurt someone else. For the Chestnut Bud types, the cycle of negative repetitive behavior can almost be an addiction. They find it difficult to take "the road less traveled" and prefer to do things the way they always have been done, even if they can see that it might lead to problems. They are creatures of habit and like to stick to a routine, afraid of anything new or different. They dislike uncharted waters and are slow to pick up on new ideas, thoughts, and philosophies. New technology, like computers, is also often avoided, preferring to do things the old way.

They are usually unable to learn the lessons of life and, subsequently, might appear to be childish or immature, even when they are old. It can almost appear that although their body has grown old, their mind is stuck at a young age and not able to progress beyond that point. This can sometimes happen if a child's parents do not want them to grow up and always want them to be their little boy or girl. An impressionable child who wants to please his or her parents can respond to this by always being a "child." Sometimes a traumatic experience during adolescence or the fear of growing up and facing responsibility can lead to a person remaining immature.

Remedy Effects

Chestnut Bud is an excellent remedy for helping people learn from experience. It can help them acknowledge their mistakes and shortcomings, and develop the courage to change themselves for the better. Rather than sticking their heads in the sand and hoping things will change by themselves, this remedy helps develop the intention and commitment to uproot bad habits and learn to live in a more balanced, creative, spontaneous, and mature manner. It empowers people to take responsibility and control over uncontrolled and negative repetitive behavior.

Chicory

Cichorium intybus

Overprotective; mothering; smothering

Chicory people simply care too much. They are over-bearing and find it difficult to give others who they care for the space to breathe. They are overprotective and often instill in their children that the world is a danger-ous place and that they need their protection. They gain a great deal of satisfaction from caring for others, strongly identifying themselves with this role to the extent that if they have no one to care for, they feel lost and often worthless.

Because of these traits, they often have difficulty in letting go of others and experience great distress when those they care for are in any kind of danger. They can dread the future if they know that those they care for will have to leave at some point. For example, the Chicory parent will not look forward to his or her chil-dren leaving home, especially if they are moving far away. As this time approaches, they will become more and more clingy and controlling, which often has the effect of making the children want to move out sooner or even farther away.

They like to organize and manage others and are gen-erally most content when in the family environment, receiving respect and reverence as the patriarch or matri-arch. They like to be in a position of authority and enjoy giving their advice and opinions, although they find it difficult if others reject this advice or go against it. They often have very strong emotional ties with family and friends and, consequently, feel a great, almost unbearable loss if someone dies or a special relationship ends. They find it difficult to let go, and others can find this emotional glue quite stifling and choking.

In extreme cases, they can be quite manipulative and even nasty if the person they want to control does not play the weak, needy role. They might become angry or sulky and try to control the person by making he or she feel guilty for not needing them. They might say things like, "You just use me," or "After all I've done for you, this is how you treat me."

Chicory children are likely to be manipulative of their siblings and parents' friends. They are clingy and demand constant love and attention. They can also be overly possessive of friends and toys. It is quite common to see a Chicory child and a Centaury child in the same family.

Some Chicory people may not appear to be overly controlling but have deep emotional attachments to people. They may even stay in a relationship that is obviously dying or damaging, because they have such a strong emotional need for companionship, finding it too hard to let go.

Remedy Effects

The positive Chicory type is loving, caring, and protective in a healthy way. This remedy promotes these qualities and allows people to feel secure enough in themselves to allow others the freedom to make their own decisions and go their own way in life, without fear of offending or worrying the Chicory type. This is a wonderful remedy to help people let go of their possessive nature and need for others.

Clematis

Clematis vitalba

Dreamy; sleepy; forgetful; always
thinking about the future

Clematis people appear to be living in a little world of
their own. A fantasy world where everything is as it
should be. No problems, no hassles, no worries. They
like to take things slowly and at their own pace. They
do not like to be pressured into quick decisions as they
easily get confused and cannot think clearly, especially
under stress. They are often absent-minded, forgetting
appointments, and mislaying keys, which can get on
others' nerves. When they feel that others are getting
irritated, they panic and become more disoriented.
Many Clematis types have a poor sense of direction,
and although they are often creative and sensitive, they
are not practical or very reliable in a crisis.

Their dreamy state of mind is usually dwelling on
happy fantasies of how they would like things to be in
the future. The obvious distinction between this and the
dreamy Honeysuckle type is that the latter tends to
dwell on the past. Although Clematis types like to have
something to look forward to and long for happier
times, they do not do much to bring these events about.
They might fall in love with someone from afar and
daydream about how wonderful it would be to be with
that person, but they may be too afraid of doing anything about it as the reality might not live up to the
dream. They also see those they do fall for in an overly
rosy light and cannot believe that they are anything but

perfect. Even if the one they love is obviously treating them badly, they may choose to ignore this or convince themselves that things will get better in the future. They are often heartbroken.

They tend to lack interest in the present, avoid real-life situations, and do not like talking about subjects that challenge their reality, especially subjects like illness and death. Their fantasy world feels safer than the world outside and is within their control. They do not like real life, preferring their own inner world where everything is rosy. Unfortunately they miss out on so much in life because of this. They often lose track of the conversation, forgetting what they were saying, and easily become bored or distracted since they lack the ability to concentrate for any length of time.

Remedy Effects

Clematis helps dreamy people wake up and smell the coffee, bringing them into the present. It gives them the confidence and courage to look at the world and themselves with honesty and clarity. There is often a strong physical change to their appearance after taking the remedy. They look more alert, alive, and "present." People who need this remedy usually report that everything seems clearer and more vivid. Their senses become sharper and their minds less dull and dreamy. People who suffer from fainting or vertigo can benefit greatly from using Clematis. It is also useful to combat the side effects of drugs that leave a person feeling dull and dreamy.

Crab Apple

Malus pumila

Feeling dirty and unclean

This is the cleansing remedy for those who feel they are not clean in some way, as if they are infected, sullied, or used. This feeling may follow a physical cause like disease, or being affected by some kind of pollution or toxic substance. The sufferer still feels that they are not clean, even after vigorous washing.

These feelings may also arise after spending time with another person who they mistrust or, in extreme cases, makes their flesh crawl. Perhaps this person was in the Crab Apple type's car and, even after a few days, they can still sense the person's presence, leaving the space unclean or polluted in some way.

Sometimes at the end of a relationship, when one person leaves another, their presence is still felt, especially if they lived together. If this presence is unwelcome or causes painful memories, Crab Apple can help people to feel fresh, clean, and free from the sense of another person's negativity, especially if it leaves them feeling soiled or used.

Crab Apple types easily feel contaminated and are often overly cautious about germs and infections. They may go to great lengths to avoid any kind of potentially infecting situation. They have almost acute standards of cleanliness that others must also conform to if they are to remain friends. They will go out of their way to avoid "dirty" people, and the thought of shaking hands and hugging such a person would almost make them sick. They are very "house proud"; their bathrooms and toilets are spotless. They expect others to have high standards, too. For example, they will only eat out if they are sure the restaurant is exceptionally clean.

In extreme cases, Crab Apple types are obsessive-compulsives, and their habits of cleanliness and avoiding dirt have taken over their lives. Everything has to be clean, and the thought of being in an unclean environment or of having to touch something that might be unclean is too much for them to bear. Although they are rare, Crab Apple children do not like to play outside or in any situation that might involve getting dirty, like a game. Crab Apple parents are always washing their children's hands, too.

Crab Apple is also indicated when people do not like themselves. They really dislike their appearance and, in severe cases, actually loathe themselves for being who they are or looking like they do. They are overly concerned with minor annoyances and easily distracted by them. If they have a cut or a minor skin problem, they may constantly pick, scratch, or look at it. They might easily get irritated by minor things and blow them out of proportion. They can also feel disgusted about basic bodily functions, the naked body, sex, illness, old age, and death.

Remedy Effects
This remedy helps Crab Apple types put things into perspective and develop a wise and balanced view on

life, instead of nit-picking and being distracted by minor annoyances. It helps people who feel dirty or used gain freedom from the agitation that accompanies the feelings of contamination, helping them feel clean physically and mentally. It enables them to relax and feel good about themselves as they are, without having to try to change their appearance or turn to external support to fulfill their inner needs.

Victims of rape or assault often feel that they are unclean, that they can still feel their assailant's presence on their body. Crab Apple can help these people begin to feel free of the other's influence.

Elm

Ulmus procera

Overwhelmed by responsibility

Elm people are capable people, usually occupying positions of authority or responsibility. They enjoy the challenge and feeling that they are doing something useful and successful. However, from time to time, they feel the pressure of responsibility is overwhelming and can become so great that they feel they cannot go on. This is often only a temporary period of self-doubt, and they usually pull through. Although there is a danger that if they experience some additional problems during one of these periods, they may believe that their confidence and ability to deal with pressure will never return. Consequently, they may make major decisions to change jobs or end relationships that they later regret when they feel stronger and more able to cope again.

When they are under pressure, they feel they are dealing with too many issues at once. They become confused because of this stress and feel that they are losing their grip on things. This can make them feel quite low as they like to feel in control and reliable, and they like others to think so, too. Consequently, they may not like asking for help when they really need it, preferring to carry on, even if things start to go wrong. Again, this can cause them to lose their normally sound judgment and make wrong decisions, becoming a little absent-minded and even forgetful.

They are usually unaware of the build-up of stress until it is too advanced or until someone tells them to take it easy or get help. The build-up of pressure can leave them feeling panic-stricken and at a loss for what to do. They may even feel like they are going to breakdown in some way. Because they are so conscientious, they will often push themselves to the limit before giving in to problems or asking for help. They may feel guilty about letting others down or looking weak in a competitive environment.

Remedy Effects

Elm promotes mental calmness, inner strength, and resourcefulness. It reduces their sense of pride so they find it easier to ask for help and not fear appearing weak. It helps them put their problems in perspective, and they are more able to prioritize and organize their time so that things get done. Elm encourages clear, rational, and methodical thought patterns and dispels confused and stressful minds. This remedy empowers the patient with self-confidence, inner strength, mental clarity, and emotional stability.

Gentian

Gentiana amarella

Despondency; despair; discouragement

Gentian is the remedy for people who give up easily when they experience any difficulty or setback. They are inclined to feel that there is no point in going on and they stop trying. They often have good intentions at the start of a project, and they are never short of good ideas, but they become easily discouraged when things don't go according to plan, or there is a series of minor setbacks.

They are creative and quick to learn, adapting to new situations easily, but they have difficulty with commitment. They do not like having to do too much work and tend to shy away from long-term plans, which they find daunting. In extreme cases, they live in a kind of childish fantasy world. They often have great plans for the future, but when the time comes to act, they usually find an excuse or diversion from having to see their ideas through.

Their energy is quickly depleted at the thought of having to do something they do not want to do, and they will try to put these things off and forget about them. This only makes it worse for them when they have to finally fulfill a promise or commitment, which at the outset seemed like a good idea.

Generally, Gentian is a good remedy for anyone who suffers any kind of setback like failing an exam, missing out on a promotion or new job, or relationship problems. Anything that causes a loss of faith in their own

abilities to succeed fills the mind with doubt and the
sufferer is left without the self-confidence to continue.

Remedy Effects

Gentian restores hope and confidence in their abilities
to achieve whatever they wish. In the face of failure,
they become less easily defeated and more inclined to
try again. This remedy encourages commitment and
perseverance in the face of adversity. It helps rid the
mind of negative self-doubt and discouragement. It lifts
the "heavy heart" and gives people the will to succeed.

Gorse

Ulex europaeus

Deep despondency and despair

Gorse is indicated whenever people are so depressed that nothing will comfort them or lift them out of their despondency. Gorse differs from Gentian in that Gentian types will tend to get better after a short time of self-doubt, so their condition is not considered severe. Gorse types, if left to their own devices, will tend to get worse and even more withdrawn. They are almost drowning in despair, as if nothing can be done to help them.

Gorse types often feel there is no hope for them; that they have reached the end of the line. The atmosphere that surrounds the Gorse person is very heavy, almost black. There is a definite sense that there is no hope to even try, and that the battle was lost long ago. When they are ill, they do not try to get better or think positively. They give in to whatever difficulty they are experiencing and sometimes do not expect to get well at all. If they do try some form of treatment, they do not expect it to work. They rarely concern themselves with how their attitude is affecting others. Consequently, they are quite hard to care for as the caregiver receives little gratitude but many complaints and comments like, "It's not worth it," "What's the point," or "Nothing and no one can help me now."

If someone experiences a series of setbacks, then the Gentian state, if not treated, can turn into the Gorse state. Again, whereas the Gentian state might last for a few hours or days, the Gorse condition is more likely to last for weeks and months if untreated. It is like an advanced, persistent Gentian condition.

Remedy Effects

Because the condition is so severe, the transformation that takes place, if the person can be persuaded to try the remedy, can be remarkable. They can quickly regain hope and start to believe that the future may hold some interesting possibilities. They become aware of how despondent they were and how this must have had a negative effect on friends and family. Consequently, they feel sorry for the way they had been acting and make an effort to be more positive, even in the face of continuing difficulties. This remedy brings increased vitality and the wish to improve.

Heather

Calluna vulgaris

Self-obsessed; talkative; dislikes being alone

Heather types like to be listened to. They like the sound of their own voice, and the more people that hear it the better. They especially like to talk about their worries, problems, ailments, or anything concerning their own affairs or those of family and friends. Usually their underlying motivation is to gain and keep the attention of others. They try to control the conversation and constantly bring it back to their own problems. They can be quite tiring and draining people. They are physical people, expressing themselves with arm gestures and loud exclamations. They will often touch others during a conversation to keep their attention and to express emotion.

Since they are generally not good listeners, they easily get bored and frustrated with other people's conversations, especially if the topic is about something that doesn't involve them or about which they know little. They tend to jump in before the other person has finished talking and use some small point of the conversation as an excuse for them to start talking again. When two Heather types meet and converse, they either get along like a house on fire or they quickly form an unfavorable opinion of each other.

They often find it difficult to empathize with others and tend to avoid people who make them feel uncomfortable. They are good at giving advice, but the advice they give is usually not very good. They will talk to

anyone and have no problem making friends and social-
izing. However, they dislike being on their own with no
one to talk to. If they have to spend time alone, they will
turn on the television or radio, sing, or try to phone
someone—anything but silence. They do not like peace
and quiet; it makes them uncomfortable and fidgety.
Although they like talking about themselves, they tend
to shy away from conversation that is moving toward
deep, meaningful, and possibly emotional subjects that,
again, make them feel uncomfortable and out of their
league. Their talkative, almost overconfident front often
hides an inner loneliness. As a result of these self-
absorbed talkative traits, people tend to avoid them,
leaving them feeling lonelier.

Remedy Effects

This remedy helps people take more interest in the welfare of others. They become more relaxed with themselves and actually learn to enjoy spending time alone.
This remedy is also effective whenever someone has
become absorbed in their own affairs to the exclusion of
all else. It helps them see that there is a world outside of
their problems and ailments. Heather brings them out
of this self-obsession and helps the sufferer take their
mind off themselves and come out into the world.

Holly

Ilex aquifolium

Strong negative emotions like envy,
suspicion, and revenge

Holly is the remedy for combating heavy negativity in
the form of hatred, envy, and rage. Sufferers cannot
help themselves. They are possessed by these emotions
that eat at their peace of mind and leave them seething
with negativity. The Holly state often arises when
someone has been emotionally hurt, such as being lied
to or cheated on. They find it difficult to think clearly
and may actually fantasize about revenge and how good
that would feel.

Jealousy is another common emotion, with sufferers
feeling overwhelmed by the wish to be like or better
than the person who is making them jealous. It is a
childish and immature state of mind and seen fairly regularly in children. The Holly remedy is therefore very
useful to have at hand when children are learning the
lessons of growing up. It can begin as a small twinge of
jealousy or dislike for another that can slowly build over
time into something much deeper and persistent if not
nipped in the bud. This might happen if a Holly type is
forced to spend time with a person they dislike, or who
is more successful or attractive than they are. If no
attempt is made at friendship, weak negative emotions
take root and grow into strong negative minds. This is
made worse by keeping these emotions inside, which is
like watering the shoots of hatred and jealousy. The

stronger these emotions become, the greater the wish becomes to act upon them in a negative way.

Remedy Effects

Holly is a great inner healer. It relieves the mental pressure and negative emotions that build up over time. It helps people become more willing to be friendly toward those they were previously suspicious or jealous of. The obvious opposite of these heavy negative emotions is love and compassion. Holly promotes these special qualities and helps people develop a real concern for others rather than treating them with suspicion or hatred.

Honeysuckle

Lonicera caprifolium

Dreamy; nostalgic; dwells on the past

Honeysuckle types tend to spend a lot of time thinking about how things used to be—the good old days. They look at the past as being much better than the present, even if in reality things were harder. They are escapists like the Clematis types and often appear dreamy and "not all there." Many elderly people develop these traits, especially if they are physically and mentally inactive or unhappy in their old age. They dwell on the past, on happier times, and relive memories over and over again in their minds. They might be surrounded by old photographs, perhaps of their children, and this serves to keep them locked into the past. They have little interest in the present. They can become forgetful and lose their concentration easily.

What they really want to do is turn back the clock. This state of mind often arises in the bereaved as they may find it difficult to face the future without the one they love, and prefer to escape in their memories rather than make plans or live with the pain of loss in the present. In fact, anyone who is experiencing difficulties of any sort may find themselves thinking back to happier times, when life was easier and they were surrounded by good things. They may tend to repeat the same story again and again in conversation without realizing it. Something like a smell or a sound may spark off a vivid memory, and then they easily lose themselves in their dreamy reverie of the past.

This remedy is also appropriate for traumatic or unhappy memories that the sufferer cannot prevent from arising in the mind. Although they may try to busy themselves in the details of daily life, whenever they stop to rest or lie down to sleep, they cannot prevent their minds from returning to whatever unpleasant experiences they have had in the past. They may relive these events over and over again, even dream about them. This can be very exhausting, and they become troubled and worried that they will never escape or come to terms with what has happened to them. They may regret past mistakes and constantly think about what they should have done.

Remedy Effects

Honeysuckle, like Clematis, helps people "wake up" and be more alive. It gives them strength to face the present and hope that the future will be good. They become less drawn toward the past and more interested in the present and what is going on in the world around them. It helps them let go of traumatic memories and come to terms with an unhappy past. Honeysuckle enables them to put past events into context rather than blowing them out of proportion and feeling that they will never be free of the effects. Honeysuckle is often suitable for sufferers of post-traumatic stress disorder. It helps them to learn from the past without being controlled by it.

Hornbeam

Carpinus betulus

Lack of enthusiasm; weariness

Hornbeam is indicated for the person who feels tired and weak at the thought of having to do something he or she does not want to do. It is the remedy for that "Monday morning" feeling, when going back to bed is better than facing another week at work.

It can be used for many situations, such as an obligation to visit someone, having to go to a party or other social event when the Hornbeam type would prefer to stay home, or having to do mundane or menial tasks that he or she wishes someone else would do. Whenever Hornbeam people are faced with a situation they would prefer to avoid, and the thought of having to go through with it leaves them feeling tired and listless, then Hornbeam can help.

Hornbeam is not a remedy for exhaustion or fatigue due to illness or overwork. Olive would suit these symptoms instead. Hornbeam is more relevant when the thought of what lies ahead leaves sufferers feeling mentally, emotionally, and, sometimes, physically weak, lacking "get up and go." Often sufferers will procrastinate and try to put things off as long as possible, but the task or situation they are avoiding plays on their minds. The thought of finally going through with what they have to do grows out of proportion the longer they leave it. Often they find that when they finally get around to it, things are not nearly as bad as they thought they might

be. There is also a great sense of relief when they have finished, and their strength and enthusiasm quickly return.

Remedy Effects

Hornbeam is the remedy for regaining enthusiasm,
strength, and taking a greater interest in life. It can be
helpful for those who have obligations and duties that
they would rather not do. Sometimes when we are caring for others, we may feel that it is becoming a chore
and that we are losing interest in the person's welfare,
feeling sapped of strength and interest. Hornbeam can
be of help at such times. This remedy can also benefit
children, such as the thought of having to go to school,
do homework, or join a sports team.

Impatiens

Impatiens glandulifera

Impatience; irritation; frustration

Impatiens is indicated for those people who are quick in thought and deed. They do not suffer fools gladly and become easily irritated when others are doing things too slowly or holding them back, making them wait in some way. They easily lose their temper and are prone to speak in haste and repent at leisure. They often prefer to work on their own without the interference of others, and they like to get things done quickly and efficiently.

Impatiens types do not like standing in line, sitting in traffic, or waiting for service. They think that everyone else should be as efficient and swift as they are. They are often quick learners and intelligent, although sometimes they get uptight if they cannot get their head around a problem. If they do ask for help, they expect it to be straight to the point. They can appear unfriendly and brusque when, in fact, they might be feeling happy and relaxed.

Sometimes they find it difficult to relax or sit for any length of time. If they watch television, they like to channel hop. A movie has to really grab their attention to keep them watching all the way through. They do not sleep in, preferring to be active and athletic—in a sense, they are addicted to activity. They find illness and disability hard to deal with and are not the best of patients. They get easily bored with others if the conversation is not stimulating; they might try to finish another person's sentences, become edgy and fidgety, or try to leave when the opportunity arises.

Remedy Effects

The Impatiens remedy helps people relax and take life a little more slowly. They become less manic and more aware of how enjoyable life is when lived at a more leisurely pace. They often begin to notice things that they did not before, like how beautiful trees are and how the seasons change. They have more time and patience with others and become more approachable and pleasurable to know. This remedy will benefit any person who is experiencing a period of tense irritability and impatience, such as during illness, while waiting for the results of an exam or medical test, or while under any kind of stress.

Larch

Larix decidua

Lack of confidence

Larch types lack confidence in their own abilities to succeed in a situation when, in fact, they are usually capable people. They lack the belief to make the most of their abilities. Unfortunately, they miss out on many opportunities in life because of this, and often mull over in their minds how things might have been if they had only done more or had more faith in themselves.

They tend to stand back and allow others, often less capable than themselves, to move ahead of them in life, and then they look at these people moving on and think, "I could have done that." Consequently, they can become quite lonely, resentful, and full of regret later in life, although these states of mind should be treated with different remedies.

They have a definite lack of self-reliance, and they are quite happy to let others do things for them if others are willing. They do not have strong vitality or a spontaneous nature and prefer to take life as it comes rather than go out into the world and see what they can achieve. They are often afraid of failure and prefer not to try rather than run the risk of failing. They tend to hold back rather than engage in life; they watch life rather than participate. Consequently, they do not learn much from life, and while their friends and contemporaries are growing, learning, and moving forward, they tend to sit back and let things pass. Sometimes they have a sudden awakening later in life as they realize time is passing by and they have not done much with their lives.

Remedy Effects

Larch helps people develop faith and confidence in themselves. It helps them to become more self-reliant and develop the wish to plunge into life with courage and boldness. They no longer sit on the sidelines but wish to be a major player and find out what life has to offer. After taking this remedy, some Larch types may make major life-changing decisions, like looking for a new career, moving house, or developing new relationships. It can almost seem like they have been reborn, catching up on lost time.

Mimulus

Mimulus guttatus

Fear of known things

Mimulus is for the shy, quiet types who tend to avoid confrontation and like to lead a peaceful life. The expression "quiet as a church mouse" comes to mind. They are sensitive people who readily take an interest in others' problems as long as they are not too difficult or challenging. They do not have a strong constitution and easily become nervous or worried, even about the smallest things. They are sometimes so shy that they avoid talking to others whenever possible. They do not like crowds and social gatherings and especially dislike loud, confident, aggressive, or boastful people. Their heart sinks if they find they cannot avoid speaking to such a person. They are very polite and also find it difficult to say no and, consequently, can be easily intimidated and taken advantage of. This might sound similar to the Centaury type; the main distinguishing trait is that Mimulus is more for shyness, timidity, and fear of know things. Centaury is more for those who are more willing servants and easily influenced by others.

They may blush or stammer during conversation and, especially, in the presence of the opposite sex or people they do not know well. Although they may be romantic, they rarely have the confidence to go and talk to someone they find attractive. They are very self-conscious and easily embarrassed, and do not like to draw attention to themselves. The thought of having to speak to a crowd of people would leave them feeling sick with fear. They would never make a fuss in public, and if they were given a bad meal in a restaurant, they would rather eat it than send it back. During illness they tend to keep quiet and do not like the attention of those they do not know. They may even put off going to see a doctor for fear of having to speak about a personal problem.

Mimulus is also the remedy for any kind of known fear, for example, fear of public speaking, the dark, spiders, heights, traveling, poverty, death, or illness.

Remedy Effects

This is the remedy for courage. This remedy gives timid, shy, and quiet types the confidence and inner strength to speak for themselves. It enables them to feel confident and not be intimidated by others. They are more able to speak their mind when necessary and less withdrawn from the world. It is helpful to take this remedy before any situation that might be worrisome for them, such as before an interview, exam, or any confrontational situation.

Mustard

Sinapis arvensis

Depression that descends and lifts quickly

Mustard is one of the remedies for depression. Not for long-term clinical depression, but for the depressive mind that descends quickly, like a heavy cloud, over the sufferer. When in the middle of this depression, it seems that it might last a long time, and there is a feeling that there is no light at the end of the tunnel. All is lifeless, pointless, and gray. Sometimes they may have no strong feelings, good or bad, about anything, just a kind of mental and emotional dullness and lack of joy. This state of mind can lift as quickly and mysteriously as it came, although it can often last for weeks and sometimes months. It may descend and lift in unpredictable cycles during this time.

It almost seems like the sufferer is two people: the normal one and the one that appears during the periods of depression. Although a series of stressful events can spark off a period of Mustard depression, there is generally no specific cause. They may not be able to actually find a reason why they feel so unhappy. It just seems as if unhappiness has suddenly arisen from within, and they cannot do anything but wait until it naturally lifts. In fact, they may say something like, "I don't know why I feel like this, I have everything I could want."

Like most people who suffer from clinical depression, they may experience other classic symptoms like sleeplessness, oversleeping, headaches, bad dreams, lack of vitality and sex drive, and general loss of interest in life. However, unlike long-term depression, all these symptoms disappear quickly when the cloud of depression lifts.

Often the depression can be felt as an emotional block, usually in the heart area, like a heavy weight on the heart. Sufferers may actually stoop or slouch forward because of this. If they have such periods of depression on a regular basis, they will often know how to do deal with them and may have developed the understanding that given time they will pass. If they are experiencing it for the first time, it can be worrisome to them and, especially, to friends and family who may not know what to do.

People who suffer these symptoms can lose hope that anything might help them. They may be afraid that if they cannot learn to control their depression, then they might lose their partner or job.

Remedy Effects

This remedy can bring happiness and joy to these people. It helps to lift the cloud of depression and fills them with hope. They are no longer at the mercy of their own dark side, and they have found a real ally and effective cure for their problem.

Oak

Quercus robur

Strong, steady, reliable type

Oak types often appear rock steady and reliable. They are regarded as people who "never let the side down" and can always be relied on to be there when needed. People often turn to them in times of trouble, and they never appear to be shaken or stirred by stressful events.

They tend to take life at their own pace and are not easily influenced by changing fashions and fads. Sometimes they do not like change, and they might stay in the same house, job, or relationship for years. Consequently, they may appear to be boring to others and lack creativity and spontaneity. They may feel a strong sense of duty and responsibility to others, so much so that they might take on too much work or agree to help others even when they actually need to rest themselves.

They generally have great stamina and staying power. They tend to never give up, and when they have set themselves a goal, they will keep on trying at a steady, almost relentless pace until they achieve what they set out to do. They do not give in when the going gets tough, and they can carry on even in the face of adversity. When ill they will struggle on with their duties and are rarely known to take time off of work or complain that they are being worked too hard. Unfortunately, this can be their downfall as they do not know when to stop. Like an ox pulling a plow, when they get their head down, they just keep on going. Eventually, if this carries on, they will lose their renowned strength and might become frustrated and unusually emotional. Often they fear losing their usually good health and strength.

Remedy Effects

Oak is the remedy for strength, determination, and commitment. It can help develop the staying power that is sometimes needed to see people through a long illness or a mentally and physically sapping long-term problem. For Oak types, it can help renew strength, but, more importantly, it can help them see that they are not indestructible, and that they need to rest sometimes; that hard work is not the answer to every problem. It also helps them develop sensitivity, gentleness, and thoughtfulness that they sometimes lack.

Olive

Olea europaea

Physical and mental exhaustion

Olive is the remedy for extreme fatigue. Sufferers feel so tired and run down that they cannot go on and want to give up. They feel that their energy and strength have all but gone, and that they have nothing in reserve. Olive can be used by anyone who feels tired and depleted after dealing with a stressful event. This state of exhaustion may follow a long period of illness where sufferers have had to put up with a lot of physical and mental pain or stress. If it seems that things are not going to improve, then the thought of facing the future makes them feel even weaker.

Olive is *not* a type remedy, although some people are more prone to giving away their time and energy to others in an unskillful way that often leaves them feeling they have nothing left to give. Instead, this remedy is helpful for caregivers who feel they have given everything to the person they are looking after and all their energy is sapped. Sometimes they even feel drained of love and concern for the patient. This indicates other remedies as well, such as Impatiens, Willow, and Holly, depending on how individuals do react to such a situation.

Olive is also excellent for people who push themselves too hard—overachievers and workaholics. The type remedy for these people will be different when they do push themselves too far for too long (perhaps Vervain, Impatiens, Elm, or Rock Water), then Olive can help them regain their strength and vitality.

Often those who could benefit from Olive have lost much of their sense of joy or love for life. They have had to deal with so much for so long that they have become less than half the person they once were. The weariness that responds well to the Olive remedy is different from the Hornbeam type. Olive is caused by overwork or overexertion whereas Hornbeam people cannot find the energy or enthusiasm to even begin the task at hand.

Remedy Effects

When the remedy is taken, there is often a quick improvement, and the sufferer can be seen to visibly grow in vitality and energy. A sparkle returns to their eyes and the body becomes less heavy and burdened with fatigue. As with all the remedies, Olive can be taken as a preventative cure when any physically or mentally strenuous project is undertaken, such as times of intense study and concentration, or when working overtime in a physically demanding job for long periods. Olive helps to restore and replenish vitality and energy.

Pine

Pinus sylvestris

Guilt; self-blame

Pine is the remedy for people who are always blaming themselves, sometimes for things that are obviously not their fault. They tend to be hard on themselves, and their thought patterns often take on a quality of self-punishment. They often do not feel good enough and may feel that a sense of guilt is a good thing. These people often come from strict backgrounds, sometimes quite religious. They may have been taught to believe from an early age that taking pleasure in the good things in life is bad and even sinful.

They may find it difficult to relax, and their strong standards and opinions about what is wrong or sinful may surface as revulsion of anything to do with love and sex. They may feel these emotions and urges but then try to ignore them or keep them within. If they do allow their minds to wander to such thoughts, they may feel guilty, and that they are dirty or bad. Pine types also tend to apologize too much. If they bump into someone, they say they are sorry many times or say, "It was my fault, I should be looking where I'm going."

They feel they are to blame when things go wrong. They may say things like, "I should have seen it coming," or "If only I'd done things differently this wouldn't have happened." They even blame themselves when things go wrong for others. They feel that they could have helped more or prevented them from making a mistake. The classic Pine type is the overly concerned parent who blames him or herself for all the mistakes the children make in life.

Remedy Effects

Pine helps sufferers free themselves from the constraints of their painful and controlling guilt. It helps them to stop apologizing to the world for who they are and feel good about themselves. It also helps them to see that they are not bad or degenerate, and that they need to love themselves and accept the good and the bad aspects of their personality. They need to fully accept the fact that they have a dark side before they can learn to work with it and transform it. Anyone who experiences guilt for something they feel they shouldn't have done can benefit from the Pine remedy. It may have happened long ago or more recently, but if they are holding these feelings, Pine can help them let go and find some mental peace and freedom from these self-destructive emotions. Pine is the remedy to combat self-reproach and remorse.

Red Chestnut

Æsculus carnea

Fear for the welfare of others

The Red Chestnut remedy is ideal for people who feel fear or great concern for the welfare of others. In extreme cases, this is not a healthy compassionate concern, but more of a selfish feeling based on the fact that the Red Chestnut type only feels at peace when those they love are at not risk from anything. They can be very overprotective parents, always saying, "Be careful," or "Don't run so fast, you might fall." When their children are playing, they often check on them every few minutes to see if they are safe. In their minds they may run through all the things that might happen to their child if they are not there to protect and guide them. Even when their children are grown up, they may always want to know they are safe and well. They may constantly ask, "Are you eating well?" and "Are you keeping warm?" They also expect to be kept informed on how things are going, and if someone doesn't phone for a while, they become worried and fretful. The children of Red Chestnut types may lose their self-confidence and learn to see the world as a dangerous, threatening place.

They become easily worried for others' safety, which can become acute at times of change, for example, when, for the first time, a child is going to school, or staying away from home, or leaving home. They find it difficult to watch anything where another person is doing something dangerous or physically challenging, like rock climbing or a high-wire act.

They may even lose sleep and develop symptoms of severe stress or trauma worrying about the welfare of people they love. An extreme case would be when a loved one is missing, and the sufferer is distraught with worry and constantly runs through all the dreadful possibilities of what may have happened to them.

Remedy Effects

This remedy works well to bring peace to a fearful mind, when the generally unfounded fear is for the welfare of others. It helps these worriers put their fears into perspective and not concern themselves with unnecessary worrying or fearful imaginings. Red Chestnut also helps these people to stop fretting and fussing over others. They are not as selfish or possessive as the Chicory type, and they tend to be more sensitive to the needs of others, and less controlling.

Rock Rose

Helianthemum nummularium

Extreme fear; terror

Rock Rose is not a type remedy, but it is used for occasional situations of extreme fear. The fear so grips sufferers that they are almost paralyzed and sometimes cannot even talk about what happened or what they are afraid of. It is definitely not nervousness or fear like the Mimulus or Aspen state. This is a much more severe and deep-seated fear.

This remedy can be helpful after a nightmare, when the person is gripped by terror or the belief that his or her life might be in danger. Children who awake from frightening dreams also find relief from using Rock Rose. Any real-life situation that creates terror can call for this remedy, for example, after a serious car crash, being attacked, or falling (vertigo). Just the fear of these things happening can also be treated with Rock Rose if the fear is extreme. If not, then Mimulus is the right remedy to choose. For example, some people are so afraid of heights, flying, or undergoing surgery that they would almost prefer to die than face these terrifying events.

There is often a feeling of panic when this remedy is relevant. The sufferer may not be able to think clearly and the mind seems to "lock," and they become incapable of action or of dealing with the situation rationally. They are like a deer caught in the headlights of an oncoming car. The sufferer may physically shake with fear, and stammer and sweat.

Remedy Effects

This remedy is wonderful for calming the mind and body. It helps those in great fear feel more able to cope and gain control again. It calms the nerves, releases tension, and brings rational thought to the mind. It also prevents extreme fear from arising before any potentially stressful experience. It can also be useful to combat nightmares.

Rock Water

Aqua petra

Strict, high, almost severe standards

People that fit the Rock Water type are very hard on themselves. Whatever their vocation or interests in life, they take them seriously—too seriously. They can almost be fanatical about whatever they are interested in. If they like sports or outdoor pursuits, they will set excessively hard goals and often push themselves too far trying to achieve them. They like to have a set routine to stick to, even if it causes them pain or distress. They do not like to feel weak or incapable and do not like others to think this either, so they will push themselves, sometimes beyond their limits, so as not to appear to fail.

Their high and harsh standards also manifest as mental and emotional rigidity. They find it difficult to express their emotions and prefer to keep them in or work them out at the gym. They may live a military-style life even if they are not in the armed forces and might expect others to "fall in line." They like to run a tight ship, and if they are the head of the family, they find it difficult to tolerate laziness or shoddiness in themselves or others. They tend not to openly criticize or convert others, but try to lead by example. When they have spare time, they prefer to do something useful and do not like loafing or just taking it easy.

They might be very religious or have high moral standards, and if they feel they are not living up to these standards, or have strayed from the path, then they might feel the need to be even harder on themselves and raise their standards higher. They like to play the martyr and, in a strange way, actually enjoy and take personal pride in their punishing regimes and stringent lifestyles. In extreme cases, they tend to deny themselves even the simplest pleasures or luxuries, and this can lead to great physical and mental tension and unhappiness.

Remedy Effects

Rock Water helps these people relax and be less hard on themselves. It enables them to enjoy life and lower their high standards so that they can be more happy and flexible in their approach to life. It lessens their sense of self-reproach and promotes notions of acceptance toward the ways of others. It helps them see that denying themselves pleasure is not a healthy mental state, and that their urges to want such pleasures are not inherently bad. It helps them to find a healthy physical, mental, and emotional balance in life while retaining their morality.

Scleranthus

Scleranthus annuus

Quiet indecision; always changing their mind

Scleranthus, like Cerato, is a remedy for indecision, however, these personality types are quite different. While Cerato types are always asking and being swayed by the opinions of others, Scleranthus types keep their worries and concerns to themselves. They may have a problem or have to make a decision, but rather than ask for help they will mull things over in their own mind. Others may not even realize that they have a problem.

This indecision is not confined to major issues as Scleranthus types have difficulty making any kind of decision, such as what clothes to wear, what to eat, or whether to phone or write to someone. Even after a decision is made doubt remains, and they are prone to changing their minds several times before making a final decision. They can be so indecisive that they become confused; their minds spin with ideas and possibilities. They tend to think about things too much and the consequences of their actions or potential actions.

Because they keep their ideas to themselves, this adds to their problems and prevents them from benefiting from the wisdom and experience of others. Often when other people talk about or share their problems, things become clearer and solutions are more easily found, but the typical Scleranthus types cannot bear to be open and honest. Their indecision can leave them feeling quite distressed and confused, and this can easily lead them in to making a wrong decision.

This remedy is also appropriate for people who are experiencing severe mood changes, i.e., one minute happy and laughing and the next minute depressed and crying, or feeling positive and confident, then negative and defeatist. This might occur during illness or in response to long-term stress or sudden shock.

Remedy Effects

This remedy is indicated whenever there are mental and emotional fluctuations. It responds by encouraging a balanced mind and a more stable perspective on life. It helps these people be more open and gives them the inner security to share their worries with others and to know their own mind. This is the remedy for mental stability, clarity, and developing a decisive confident mind. This remedy is often very useful for travel or motion sickness.

Star of Bethlehem

Ornithogalum umbellatum

Shock

This remedy is excellent for treating people who have experienced any kind of severe shock. It might be recent or occurred many years before. The shock might be a serious accident, the death of a loved one, a burglary or other criminal act, terrible news, or a horrific or appalling sight. Sometimes it might not be an obvious or sudden shock, for example, a long-term problem like financial worries or illness, which may leave sufferers looking back on what has happened to them and feel shocked and aghast at how their life has changed.

People who need Star of Bethlehem may seem bewildered, lost, and in a daze when they talk about their problems. They might say that they feel they have been caught up in a whirlwind of problems, and that their feet have not touched the ground, saying, "I can't believe what has happened to me." This statement describes exactly how shock is experienced. It is a sense of disbelief, of being knocked sideways and not feeling "all there" as a result. In severe emergency cases, the sufferer may be shaking, unable to talk, or lose consciousness.

This remedy can greatly help those experiencing grief. It can release trapped or bottled up emotions that the shock of the loss has kept within, relieving the sadness and feelings of loss. Shock may be delayed, for years even, and any remedy that is being given for a condition arising from a shocking or deeply stressful event should include Star of Bethlehem.

Remedy Effects

Star of Bethlehem brings calmness and relief from the grip of shock. It enables sufferers to let go of the stressful event and makes it less dominant and significant in their mind. This remedy promotes a more realistic and stable mental and emotional state and brings clarity, perspective, and peacefulness to the mind.

Sweet Chestnut

Castanea sativa

Severe mental distress; anguish

Sweet Chestnut is the remedy for extreme mental and emotional anguish. When this remedy is indicated, sufferers are usually so distraught that they cannot be consoled or comforted. They are in a state of severe psychological pain and distress, either openly manic or introverted and desperately trying to control the mind. There is a sense of great despair and loss of hope, and they feel that no solution to their problems can be found, as if there is no light at the end of the tunnel, and that all the future holds is more suffering.

Often they feel desolate inside or so sad and unhappy that they physically feel heavy or empty within. They may feel so awful that they actually wish to die, but tend to believe that even death would not release them from their distress.

Sometimes they feel stretched to the limits of their mental endurance, and that if some relief is not found soon, they will simply break under the strain. There may be a palpable sense of the end approaching—of doom, destruction, or annihilation.

The main symptom of Sweet Chestnut types is this sense of inner destruction and desolation coupled with a belief that there is no hope for a brighter future. For example, this remedy might be appropriate for someone who is facing the prospect of a long-term or life-threatening illness, living life without a loved one, or trying to cope with the effects of famine, war, or some other major conflict or disaster. This remedy might also be appropriate when a person cannot avoid living or working in a place he or she greatly dislikes or fears, when the person's unhappiness is so great that the time he or she has to spend in that place seems to stretch far into the future.

Remedy Effects

Sweet Chestnut can have a wonderfully calming and healing effect on these people. The state of mind sufferers experience is so extreme that when the remedy is taken, there is a tremendous sense of relief, and they begin to feel some of the internal strain lift and dissipate. They also feel a renewed sense of hope and an improved mental attitude toward their situation. A feeling of optimism returns along with a will and resolve to approach life with a positive attitude.

Vervain

Verbena officinalis

Overenthusiasm; physical and mental strain

Vervain types are conscientious and hard working. They have high ideals and standards, and it is often their mission in life to help others see that their ways are the best. They can be evangelical and try to convert others to their way of thinking. They do this not for the sense of power or control, but because they have genuinely good intentions and wish to help others. Their boundless enthusiasm might often be for environmental, educational, political, or spiritual issues or for some other good cause. Whenever they have a chance to talk to someone about these issues, they will do their best to interest them in these worthy causes; they like to show others the way.

Vervain types often make good sales people. Their enthusiasm can be infectious and leads them to be successful in whatever field they choose. However, they can be prone to working or pushing themselves too far, and this can lead to physical and mental strain that might sometimes take the form of a nervous breakdown or other classic symptoms of stress, like depression. They can become frustrated if they feel their work is not progressing well or if problems and difficulties arise. They tend to be quick-thinking and active people, full of good ideas and good intentions.

If they do push themselves too hard or experience too many frustrating setbacks, then tension can build up within, and they can become impatient and snappy, appearing high-strung. They are definitely not plodders and sometimes find it difficult to relax and unwind.

Remedy Effects

The Vervain remedy helps people slow down and learn to accept difficulties and setbacks with a peaceful and philosophical mind. They become more accepting of others and more open and interested in their ideas and beliefs. It creates a sense of being that is relaxed and tension free. It does not dull their enthusiasm or creative energy, but simply helps them to live within their limits and learn to relax and recharge themselves regularly.

Vine

Vitis vinifera

Leaders; powerful and controlling attitude

Vine is the remedy for people who are the natural leaders in society. They are attracted to roles where they can lead and influence others. In extreme negative states, they enjoy the power and authority and like to exercise their control in a manipulative and self-centered manner. Sometimes their wish for power, dominance, and control is so great that they will do anything to reach a position of authority—and once there will do anything to keep it. The classic extreme Vine type is the military dictator who is feared by his subjects and servants.

The positive Vine types are excellent leaders and great examples to others. They might have a responsible job where they are in charge of a large department or company, often with many people under their influence. If they are a benevolent and kind boss, people will love them and look up to them. If they act more like a dictator, they often end up feeling lonely and separate from their employees.

Power and control is often an addiction to these people, and those close to them might find their confidence, ambition, and authority attractive and persuasive, or repulsive and childish. Either way, they often evoke strong feelings in others. They know their own minds and thrive on responsibility and challenges. They like to direct others and tell them what they can and cannot do. There is often no room for reasoning, debate, or argument, though; what the Vine type says, goes. These characteristics are often easily seen in children who like to control and command others. The gentle and willing Centaury type is often a victim of the Vine person.

Remedy Effects

The Vine remedy acts to release their need to control the lives of others and helps them channel their natural leadership qualities into more positive roles. They become more willing to listen to the opinions of others and more motivated to help others rather than use them for their own purposes. They especially become more understanding and even protective of those with a gentle disposition rather than despising weakness and sensitivity.

Walnut

Juglans regia

Easily influenced by others

Walnut is the remedy for protection. It is not generally seen as a type remedy, but some people will be more likely to use this remedy than others. The people that will most benefit from Walnut are those who are easily influenced by others during times of change, either externally or within the mind. If someone is like this most of the time, a more appropriate remedy might be Centaury.

We all experience a certain amount of nervousness or vulnerability at times of change or upheaval, and these are the indications for Walnut. Examples of when Walnut might be appropriate are when moving house, emigrating, changing jobs, receiving a promotion, getting married, having a child, or beginning a new relationship—basically any major change that leaves a person feeling a little disoriented and out of sorts. It can help cut mental and emotional ties with the past that might be holding people back and preventing them from giving their full energy to new situations and new relationships.

It can also be very helpful during those times of new beginnings in life like the change from baby to child to young adult to adult and so on, right through to retirement and the coming of old age. This remedy also prevents people from being knocked off course in life. It helps them to decide for themselves which routes to take, free from the influence of others.

Any other disturbing influence that someone may be experiencing can be combated by using Walnut. For example, someone may have to live in a city where it is noisy, dirty, or even dangerous, or in a house with other people who make him or her uneasy.

Remedy Effects

As Walnut is the remedy for protection, it can help us to keep a peaceful mind in spite of these worrying or stressful influences. If people are particularly open to the ideas and influences of others, Walnut can prevent them from being led astray and help them to judge what is right and wrong. Often children who are being bullied or persuaded to be more disruptive by strong-willed peers can be helped to stand their own ground and think for themselves. People of a spiritually sensitive nature who are troubled by negative energies or spirits can also become stronger and less vulnerable by using Walnut regularly. It can also be a useful remedy for therapists or those working in the health professions, as it helps protect the caregiver and prevents them from picking up any of the patient's "stuff."

Water Violet

Hottonia palustris

Proud; aloof; quiet

Water Violet types are seen as being proud and sometimes superior. They do not see themselves as proud, but they often do feel superior to others. They look down on those around them and see these people as being coarse or ignorant, and then feel that they are on a higher plane than the others. This can cause them to live a lonely existence, as they feel unable to open up and talk to others about their problems, unless they feel the other person is on the same high level.

They are often quiet and thoughtful people and do not like large crowds, noisy rooms, or energetic parties. They prefer their own company or that of a few well-known and trusted friends. Their natural disposition is generally positive and confident and, like the plant itself, they often stand proud and erect. Their physical movements are graceful and elegant, rarely rushed or erratic.

They try not to influence others but will give advice if asked. Generally, they prefer to watch rather than take part in life. Because they are so quiet and observant, they often see the mistakes that others are going to make before they make them. This might lead them to feel even more superior, or wanting to help others in some way, perhaps through counseling or some other quiet and thoughtful vocation. Others often think Water Violet types are wise and self-sufficient, and they often put them on a pedestal, looking up to them as an example of perfection. The egos of Water Violet types enjoy this attention, but ultimately leaves them feeling even more lonely and distant from the rest. Because of this distance and the emotional barriers, they have a strong inner need for love and affection, which their pride often prevents them from getting since they are not gregarious or naturally outgoing, shunning those who are.

Remedy Effects

Since Water Violet types tend to keep their problems within and do not find it easy to be open emotionally, unless they feel very secure, this remedy helps them develop some trust in others and also a little humbleness, which is the antidote to pride. It helps them to see that no man is an island; they are not always right and they do need others to survive. They become more approachable, friendly, and less distant and removed from life. They are able to take a more active and involved role in life without losing their quiet wisdom and thoughtfulness.

White Chestnut

Æsculus hippocastanum
Unwanted disturbing thoughts

The White Chestnut remedy is useful when a person is unable to prevent unwanted and often distressing thoughts and emotions from arising. There is a lack of mental peace, and sufferers are plagued by constant and often unfounded worries. Sometimes this condition may be more noticeable at night or when resting, when there are fewer distractions to occupy the mind. As a result of this condition, many people become tired and worn out as they find it difficult to sleep. They may also wake up frequently, and their mind automatically returns to their worrisome thoughts. The amount of mental energy they use up and the constant stress of the agitated mind can also leave them feeling confused and worn out.

Often the White Chestnut person will appear to be thinking about something else, even while in conversation, as if their mind is elsewhere. There might not necessarily be an obvious cause for their persistent worries; the mind just finds something troublesome to think about. If there has been a long period of stress and agitation, then the mind becomes so familiar with entertaining problems that it finds it difficult to let go of this habit. They may find it difficult to concentrate, and the symptoms might appear as fidgeting and restlessness.

In extreme cases, the White Chestnut state of mind is out of control. Sufferers can find no inner peace or freedom from their disturbing inner world. The White

Chestnut state, if not caught right away, can sometimes lead to more serious conditions, like the Cherry Plum or Sweet Chestnut conditions.

Remedy Effects

White Chestnut brings relief from the persistent worries that arise in the mind. It helps to establish a sense of inner peace and freedom from these mental disturbances. It also promotes an understanding of the importance of being rather than doing and thinking all the time.

Wild Oat

Bromus ramosus

Looking for direction or purpose

Wild Oat people can often seem listless, bored, and without energy. This is due to their lack of direction or purpose in life. Usually they have experienced much and have had many jobs, partners, or change of address-es, but it is as if they are still searching for something. They may become tired, disillusioned, and aimless because of their searching. It is also a mental searching. They often spend time wondering about what they should be doing with their lives but never come up with anything that really grabs them. If they do find some-thing that they think might be right for them, they will often try it for a short time and then change their minds and continue searching again.

They can be quite immature people and appear to not have grown up—a sort of adolescent adult. They may not actually want to take responsibility for their lives and instead prefer to play around and loaf, rather than find a useful occupation or career. This might show in their behavior and the ways they treat others.

However, they just have not found their vocation in life. They may have a strong wish to do something worthwhile but not know what it is. Because of this, they lose interest in life and appear lost and listless, almost like a lost soul. Their energies are dissipated, because they have no focus or direction, and there can be a feeling of despondency or dissatisfaction.

Remedy Effects

Wild Oat helps these indecisive and directionless people develop an inner maturity and find a sense of purpose in life, helping them to become responsible citizens. This remedy is also useful when someone is looking for a new direction in life but finding it difficult to clearly see what an appropriate direction might be. Whenever people are at a major crossroads in life, Wild Oat can help them to gain clarity and confidence in choosing a suitable direction. It can also help during adolescence when some young people may be reluctant to become mature and responsible adults.

Wild Rose

Rosa canina

Apathy; laziness

Wild Rose types have little interest in anything. They are lazy and prefer to do nothing rather than try to change things for the better. They are apathetic and lack interest in the welfare of others and even themselves. Extreme Wild Rose types have given up caring about anything. They feel heavy and tired, lacking energy and vitality. They are not creative or spontaneous and prefer to keep away from people who are annoying, as they disturb their wish for a quiet and easy life; although we know sometimes opposites attract.

They may often end up without a job or with one that is undemanding. They lack imagination and avoid change or any kind of disturbance to their routine, if they have one. They are not morning people and prefer to stay in bed if possible. They have no ambition to move or better themselves, but prefer to accept things as they are and drift along through life, applying as little effort as possible. They might say things like, "That's life," "That's just the way things are," or "Let's not rock the boat."

Wild Rose people are passive and give up easily. They are not defeatist but more like they cannot be bothered. If they are ill, they do not fight it but submit to the limitations it imposes. They may be emotionally flat, without strong good or bad feelings toward anything, rarely being very happy or deeply unhappy.

Remedy Effects

Wild Rose helps these people sit up and take a renewed interest in life. They become more energetic and revived from their mental and emotional dullness. A sense of spontaneity and vitality is restored, and they are more likely to make new plans and take on new projects as their wish to live life more fully gradually develops. They will still prefer to take things as they come and be philosophic about difficulties, but they will also be more able to deal with things in a positive and energetic manner.

Willow

Salix vitellina

Introspective; self-obsessed

Willow types react to difficulties and problems by becoming quiet, withdrawn, and introspective. They can be melancholic and enjoy wallowing in their own problems. This can bring others down; just being in the presence of a severe Willow type can leave another person feeling low and heavy. They tend to sap the energy of others in a way that is similar to the Heather type. While both types are self-obsessed, they differ in the way they try to gain the attention of others. Heather types are openly talkative, while the Willow types are more quiet and sulky.

Willows will dwell on their own problems and past misfortunes. The sadness they feel is strangely comforting, and there is a subtle sense of self-righteousness. They may feel resentful toward others or toward life, wondering why they have been so unfortunate. There is a definite "why me" attitude, and this is accentuated if others close to them are more fortunate or successful. They can become trapped in this cycle of self-pity, grumbling and moaning whenever they have an opportunity.

They may find it difficult to let go of the past if they are now experiencing difficulties because of it. Consequently, they find it hard to forgive and forget and can become embittered and pessimistic.

Remedy Effects

This remedy helps people emerge from their self-absorption, dwelling less on their own personal misfortunes. They become more optimistic and less caught up in their own little world of self-gratifying pessimism. They stop blaming others and life in general, and begin to look on the positive side of things. They become more interested in the welfare of others, and there is often a time of apology as they realize how selfish they have been.

Nine

Stories, Advice, and Case Studies

Many people all over the world have positive stories and experiences to share about the Bach remedies. This chapter contains a representative cross-section of those that were sent to the author upon request. These stories, some of them funny, some poignant and moving, show the versatility and effectiveness of the remedies in different situations. All of these shared experiences point to one thing: anyone can benefit from using these remedies and, with a little experience, knowledge, and a good heart, can help many others gain relief from all kinds of physical and mental difficulties.

The first few stories demonstrate the power of the well-known Rescue Remedy. These are followed by some detailed case studies and testimonies to the healing power of the other Bach remedies. (If you would like to contact any of the contributors, please write to the author.)

Fear Not

When I met her she was a wreck. The client was suddenly experiencing extreme anxiety and fear. It came upon her almost overnight and lasted about two months. She was afraid of getting in the car for fear of an accident, she was afraid her dog was going to get shot by the neighbor, she was afraid her husband would die of ulcers, and she was afraid she would lose her job. The list went on and on with known as well as unknown fears.

I made her a remedy of Mimulus, Aspen, and White Chestnut. She took the first drops and fell back on her chair. She said, "Wow!" and just sat there looking stunned. After a few moments she smiled and said, "It's gone." The fear had left her in that one dose—and it has never returned.

A different story shows the versatility of Bach's Rescue Remedy. One day I had to uproot a rather large pine tree (about seven feet tall). My neighbor didn't want it near his driveway as it blocked his view of traffic, so I transplanted it to another spot. I filled a bucket with water and added about twenty drops of the Rescue Remedy to the water. I watered the newly transplanted tree with it and also put some Rescue Remedy into a bottle of water and sprayed the tree while I talked to it, urging it to stay alive. I knew it had received a tremendous shock.

The good news is that it never showed the least sign of shock, neither wilting or looking bad in any way. It maintained its beauty as if it had always grown in its new place. I watered and sprayed it with Rescue Remedy solution for a week, then every other day for a week and it continues to thrive.

—*Haripriya Dillon*
Bach flower practitioner,
healer, naturopathic doctor, therapist

Remedy Cream to the Rescue

Two days ago while getting out of my car I sprained my ankle. That evening the pain was so intense with it throbbing and swelling, I could not apply any pressure on the foot and walking was impossible. I applied Rescue Remedy cream on the sprained area and within minutes the pain and throbbing stopped. I borrowed a wheelchair to get around the house for the evening. When I woke up the next morning I was able to walk.

Another story involving Rescue Remedy cream concerns my two-month-old daughter. When she was about three weeks old she developed what doctor's call infant acne, a red rash that covered her face. I was told the rash could last up to five months. I began applying Rescue Remedy cream and within a week the rash cleared completely.

—*Iris Chiappolini*

The Stubbed Toes

A few months after my eighteen-year-old son moved out of the house, I suddenly realized I had the entire house to myself. There was no need to keep his bedroom sitting there going to waste as he would probably never stay with me again. So, I decided to take it over, as it was the nicest room in the house, overlooking the back porch. That was just the beginning. I went rather wild moving rooms around, in a hopscotch feng shui sort of manner. My bedroom moved to his room, his bedroom moved out to the porch, and so on. With all this lifting, I needed a local handyman to help me. As I don't wear shoes in the house, he was forced by this tradition to remove his boots. We were doing quite well when suddenly he yelled out that he had stubbed his toe. I rushed over to have a look and saw that it was bleeding. I first went for the Rescue Remedy and put some in his mouth, and then put a few drops on the toe. Since it had alcohol in it, it also acted as an antiseptic. I wrapped his toe with a bandage, and he was off to work again as though nothing had happened.

About an hour went by when he stubbed his other toe. I guess he wasn't used to going barefoot while he worked. Suddenly I heard his loud masculine voice yell, "Quick! Get that painkiller. I did it again!" I had to laugh. The Rescue Remedy had worked so well with toe number one, that he thought I had given him a painkiller for it.

I've used this method on more than one stubbed toe, as I will tell you in another story.

My teenage son Janaka and his friend Andrew were playing in the backyard one afternoon. I heard a scream, and both boys rushed into the house. Janaka was limping and hopping, his face contorted in pain and shock. He was crying and moaning, quite distressed. His normal behavior was "all boy" and he wasn't a crybaby, so I knew it had to be serious. That's when I noticed his bloody toe. The nail was torn half off, and I imagined the pain to be excruciating.

I grabbed my trusty bottle of Rescue Remedy and put a few drops onto my son's toe and had him take a few drops orally. I repeated the treatment several times over the next two to three minutes. Janaka suddenly relaxed, sighed deeply, and with a silly giggle imitating a drunk said, "Wow! What's in that stuff?" He could taste the brandy preservative and thought I had given him something to drink. Andrew piped up, "Well, I want some, too!" So I joined in the fun and gave Andrew his share, too. In a few seconds the pair were laughing and running around, having already forgotten the crisis. I sat down and breathed a sigh of relief and had a few drops myself. As many times as I had used my beloved Rescue Remedy it still astonished me how quickly it can work.

The sequel to this little drama took place one month later at an evening seminar I was attending. As I walked down a poorly lit path to the area where the lectures were being held I stumbled on some loose gravel, severely stubbing my toe. A piercing pain shot through my foot causing me to yell loudly. Several people saw me stumble and immediately came to assist me. They helped me as I hopped to a nearby cabin where I sat to take the pressure off my foot.

The pain had increased two-fold by this time and it took all the control I could muster not to cry. I managed to ask if anyone had any Rescue Remedy handy. Somewhat to my surprise and good fortune a lady had a small bottle of it in her purse. She said that she always carried Rescue Remedy with her whenever she left her house. Though it was nearly empty there was enough for me to apply a few drops on my toe and take some orally. I did this several times, and remembered my son's experience with Rescue Remedy when he bruised his toe and the transformation, which seemed to occur just after the treatment. I was pleased to notice the pain in my toe subsiding and disappearing within five minutes.

The pain did not recur. I was able to walk normally to the seminar. I thought it an unusual coincidence that my son and I would both so severely stub our toes, apply Rescue Remedy, and experience immediate physical and emotional relief from the painful bruise. It saved the day for my son and it saved the night for me. Thank you, Dr. Bach, and thank you Rescue Remedy.

—*Haripriya Dillon*

A Burning Issue

I was at my parent's house in Lincolnshire looking for a place to attach the leash of my dog Bilbo's leash while we unpacked the car. My mother was unhappy at my tying the leash on a flower potholder on the wall by the door. I was in the process of trying to unhook it when he spied another dog and took off in pursuit. I, of course, was instinctively worried about pulling the potholder off the wall so I grabbed hold of the lead itself, which slithered through my left hand at a high rate of speed.

Naturally enough I burnt all four fingers, one of them right through the skin. All I had with me was the Rescue Remedy so I applied this at regular intervals during the evening (it happened in the afternoon). By the next day two of my fingers had more or less healed, the little finger that was badly scorched was considerably healed and the one that had gone through to the flesh was much better. In a couple of days they had all completely healed. I had not had personal experience of the physical healing ability of Rescue Remedy so I was almost pleased in a way that this had happened.

—*Sheila Bennett*

Sold!

On a recent trip to Hawaii I was packed like a sardine into a large airliner. Then, to top things off, a baby in the seat behind me was screaming nonstop, stretching the patience of the already overworked stewardess in my section, and I'm sure irritating the nerves of most of us sitting nearby. Suddenly I got an idea. I called the stewardess over to me and asked if she had heard of Rescue Remedy. She had not so I briefly told her about it, and asked her to see if the mother of the baby would agree to put some on the pulse points of the baby's wrists. She agreed as I explained as simply as I could about Rescue Remedy to her. There was a little hesitancy, but the screams of the baby quickly made her change her mind, and she, too, agreed it was worth the try. I then put a few drops of Rescue Remedy onto the mother's fingers, and she gently rubbed it onto the baby's little wrists. Within a few minutes the baby stopped crying and soon was fast asleep. I looked back and we exchanged smiles of relief. The stewardess, who was sixty-three years old, had worked for the airlines for forty years. We chatted awhile, and she said that in the last few years a strange phenomenon was occurring. She called it "airline rage." She said people were more irritable, impatient, surly, and angry, with an "in your face" attitude the likes of which she had never experienced before in her career. Babies cried more and longer, and the stewardesses had new challenges of coping with all of this that was beyond the call of duty. I talked to her at length about

Dr. Bach's flower essences, and suggested she keep Rescue Remedy with her at all times. Looking down on the sleeping baby she said, "Sold!"

—*Haripriya Dillon*

A Healer Abroad

Recently I had the privilege of being in the position of fulfilling an ambition of doing some voluntary work overseas. I became a team member of an organization called Healing Hands Network, a nationwide association of complementary and orthodox health care professionals dedicated to helping relieve the suffering caused by the effects of war and other disasters.

I traveled to Sarajevo in Bosnia and Herzegovina to work as a complementary therapist for two weeks. During my stay there I used the Bach Flower Remedies with some of the people I treated. I would like to share one elderly gentleman's response to the remedies.

In June 1997, I was teamed up with a doctor and translator to do some house visits. The first person I was taken to see was an elderly gentleman who looked much older than his seventy years. His name was Bosko and he was suffering from diabetes and colitis. He looked frail and frightened and was also emaciated and ill-looking. From my past experience of working as a nurse in a hospice for several years, I felt that Bosko did not have long to live. The doctor asked if I could do anything for him, as there was nothing else they could do.

It has to be remembered that although the war is over, there is still a lot of tension and "no go" areas. It was a near impossibility to have Bosko moved to hospital because of the political situation. It was therefore left to his wife, Radmila, to care for him. They had been married for over forty years and had one son who was married with one daughter. Their son was unable to come back home because it was unsafe for him to do so.

The doctor, translator, Bosko, and Radmila had absolutely no idea about the remedies or the principles of the system. The reason I chose to use the remedies was because there was nothing else that I thought was appropriate out of the therapies I practice; I also knew they would be safe to use.

It took quite a while to explain about the remedies and how they work, but time was one thing everyone seemed to have. My explanation of the remedies and the system of healing was directed at everyone. Bosko appeared to be asleep, but his wife listened intently. As one can imagine it took quite a while to explain that it was a medical doctor who had discovered the flower remedies in the 1930s and how they represented a complete system of healing for the emotional health, mood, and personality of people. What surprised me was the total faith they had in what I was saying—even the doctor. To make sure that they had fully understood what I had said I doubled-checked via the translator that the doctor would be happy for me to leave some remedies with Bosko, and that he and Radmila would be willing to use them.

I had only taken a few remedies with me and these were Rescue Remedy, Star of Bethlehem, Rock Rose, and Honeysuckle. I had not brought treatment bottles, only the concentrates due to a lack of packing space. I was taking many things from a list of things needed. During the visit Radmila supplied the information via the translator, apparently Bosko declined to take insulin for his diabetes. I am unsure why this was but I was told that each patient had to pay in full for a prescription and this was very expensive and quite often medication was not affordable.

I chose just one remedy and this was Star of Bethlehem. The reason for selecting this remedy was to address the aftereffects of the shock caused by the recent war and the continuing uncertainties, also the extreme sadness and grief of not being able to see his son, daughter-in-law, and grandchild and the distress of being so physically ill and weak. I also instinctively felt that the chosen remedy took preference over the use of Rescue Remedy. In the past I had ignored my instincts and regretted so when in actual fact it would have been the correct thing to do.

I explained to the doctor and Radmila that the reason I was leaving the Star of Bethlehem was that it would help calm Bosko and feel more at peace and less distressed. Had I taken a wider selection of the remedies with me I would have included Olive to address the apparent physical and mental exhaustion. I also toyed with the idea of including some Honeysuckle but decided against it still thinking to work with the one remedy. It was difficult to arrive at a key remedy because of Bosko's extreme weakness and most of the information was coming from his wife. I instructed Radmila to put two drops of Star of Bethlehem into a glass of water and to let Bosko take frequent sips of the prepared remedy.

I soon found out that once you had treated one family member the doctor would then ask if there was anything you could do for the patient's partner. I gave Radmila a small bottle of Rescue Remedy, instructing her how to use it.

I saw Bosko two days later and he had deteriorated further. He was falling and had several bruises to show for it. He was having a lot of diarrhea due to his colitis and was reluctant to drink fluids as he felt this made the problem worse. Emotionally he was very weak and not up to talking even to the doctor. I asked Radmila to increase Bosko's drops up to two drops in a teaspoon of water, four times a day. My reason for doing this was again instinctive, but also I was concerned that Bosko was unable to drink a full glass of water plus remedy over the course of a day. Another reason was that I remembered reading in *The Medical Discoveries of Edward Bach Physician* by Nora Weeks that Agrimony had been used hourly. This was not what I was taught, but I felt there would be no harm using the remedies this way as there really was little else I or the doctor could offer. I also spent five minutes gently massaging Bosko's feet using some lavender oil diluted in sweet almond oil as a means of comfort.

Five days later I went with the doctor to visit Radmila and Bosko. I must admit I was surprised to hear that he was still alive although I did not voice my thoughts. Radmila was at the gate to meet us with a big smile on her face and began to talk very quickly, but obviously I didn't have a clue what was being said. Once inside the bedroom it became obvious what all the excitement was about. Bosko was sitting up in bed eating popcorn and looking like a different person. We all stood looking on in amazement. Apparently he became much more responsive twenty-four hours after the last visit, his mobility was much steadier, and he had even managed to sit in the garden forty-eight hours after the last visit. The diarrhea was not as acute and Bosko was able to take more fluids. I asked Radmila to continue with the same regime of taking the Star of Bethlehem. I repeated the aromatherapy massage on Bosko's feet and was amazed to see a vast improvement to the healing of his old varicose ulcers from the last visit. Although they had not been deep open lesions there was still a degree of healing needed and I was certainly surprised to see the change in five days.

Another two days later I made my last visit to see Bosko. The improvement had been maintained and there was a definite twinkle in his eyes. When the translator told him this Bosko acknowledged he was feeling lighter and wished he could dance. He was still able to walk unaided to the bathroom and he had been out in the garden again. Also he was still eating and drinking though in very tiny amounts.

From my first visit to my last visit there had been quite a dramatic change in Bosko's emotional and also his physical health and well-being. He was now able to communicate more readily and appeared much more relaxed, calmer, and even happy. I felt it was appropriate to continue with the Star of Bethlehem but to reduce the number of times per day from four to two. I also thought it was now appropriate to include the Honeysuckle remedy to help Bosko release the unpleasant thoughts and memories he was dwelling on. I explained to Bosko and Radmila why I was leaving the extra remedy and they were pleased to continue using them. Radmila commented that she was feeling more relaxed and more able to continue with life and provide care for Bosko.

In the ideal world I would have continued monitoring Bosko's responses for a while longer, making any alterations as appropriate. This was not ideal, but at least Bosko had received the wonderful benefits of the remedies, perhaps at a time when he most needed them.

Since my return home I have heard that Bosko is still alive and although his physical condition is weakening he remains emotionally at ease. This information was given to me from a therapist who has just returned from Sarajevo. She had visited Bosko and Radmila, but in the capacity of a healer/aromatherapist.

Although I was unable to conduct Bosko's consultation directly with him and use the remedies to their full potential I feel he benefited greatly. For me it was a learning experience both personally and professionally and a humbling experience.

The people I encountered were very grateful and this experience reinforced my belief to keep it simple, listen to one's intuition, listen to the individual, and have faith.

—Serena Shepperd
Bach flower practitioner, aromatherapist,
reflexologist, bowen

Anxiety Case Study

A twenty-six year-old business administrator made an appointment with me for his feelings of anxiety. He had already tried other conventional therapies and treatments, he had taken some prescription pills in order to lower the anxiety, but these did not help.

At first he looked for books on the Bach Flower Remedies. Then, he decided to look for a professional who could help him. He saw an interview I gave on television about the Bach remedies.

He came for an interview and I explained how the remedies worked and a little of the philosophy behind them. I noticed that during the first twenty minutes of the session he kept sitting on the edge of the chair. After that, he began feeling more confident and comfortable and sat back and began to talk more openly. By the end of the interview he had decided to try the Bach remedies.

Considering his overall posture, the way he spoke, and the problems that he was experiencing I determined he was the Oak type. His anxiety consisted of trying to sustain the world on his shoulders. He was trying to complete his own education and work at the same time in order to make enough money to provide for his brother's studies as well as buy a new house for their widowed mother. We talked about lowering the level of his anxiety by using Impatiens and Oak to help him see that his obligations were not so heavy. We also discussed using Gentian to increase his faith in being able to succeed. I recommended that he take the remedies four times a day, four drops each time.

When the patient returned I noticed that he sat more relaxed than in the first interview. He told me he was feeling less anxious and not as tired anymore. He was facing problems in a natural way and he felt he could achieve his goals without great harm. We talked about the priorities of his life and we concluded that sometimes he still felt anxious because he thought he might not be able to accomplish everything. We spoke about his low self-esteem and he agreed that if we could improve this mental aspect he would feel at ease and more able to cope. The prescription this time was Larch to improve his confidence and self-esteem, Elm to relieve the feeling of being overwhelmed by his responsibilities, and Agrimony to see the truth and be open and honest about his worries. White Chestnut was also added to prevent constant worry and things mentally piling up on him.

After a month, the patient returned saying he had talked to his former therapist about the benefits of the new treatment (Bach remedies). He had greatly reduced his intake of the anxiety drug, taking the medicine every other day. By our third session he was talking about stopping taking the pills. He was feeling much more confident and even considering the possibility of a job for his brother while working to help him to buy a new house for their mother. He also said he was driving his car slower, and that now he had found time to have lunch everyday. He was very happy.

During his fourth session I prescribed Walnut for adapting to this new lifestyle, Gorse to help with his occasional feelings of deep discouragement, and Mimulus to face his difficulties with courage.

The patient's progress was wonderful. His anxiety was gone, he acknowledged how much the remedies had helped him and the weight on his shoulders had finally lifted. He now expects to buy his mother's house soon while his brother continues his education, and their finances are secure.

—*Cyana Saccomani*

A Life in Healing

My introduction to the Bach Flower Remedies was about twenty-five years ago. I had just gone through a traumatic time in my life; my marriage had come to an end, and due to the unreasonable actions of my husband, I had to give up my son. It was only my strong spiritual beliefs that sustained me.

I had by this time read *The Finding of the Third Eye*, by V. S. Alder, which confirmed the things I had already discovered myself. I learned to meditate, and then went on to form a group and began to teach meditation, helping people to make contact with their own higher consciousness or soul, this being the most helpful and spiritual thing we as "servers" can do for others.

One day I went into the local health store and, not by chance, my hand alighted on Dr. Bach's book *Heal Thyself*. This little book was for me another part of the jigsaw, another tool for helping people. I proceeded to learn the remedies and made them first for myself and then for friends and family. I was very encouraged by the results. Some years passed, during which I worked with all the tools I already had: meditation, the healing Bach Flower Remedies, and visualization. I used whichever tool that seemed most appropriate for the person I was working with, aiming to help them change their perception, remove the mental/emotional blockage, and allow the soul to flow a little stronger. Realizing, like Dr. Bach, how important the state of mind and emotions were in the healing process I added another tool to my collection and I achieved my qualification in NLP (Neurolinguistic Programming), which proved to fit in well with the therapies I already used.

At this time (fourteen years ago), the group I had formed was anxious to spread the wisdom we had gained with others. We rented a local meeting house and set up a holistic self-help and support group. We registered with various agencies and groups and began working with a steady stream of people of all ages and backgrounds with much success. Healing and the other therapies we used were a bit "way out" in those days, but they have become much more acceptable over the last twenty years. We have grown with the times and added other therapies and ways of healing and now teach self-help groups, and spiritual development, still also working one on one. The Bach remedies are an important part of my work, and have proved to be most useful, whatever stage of development people are at.

Although we must not put people into compart-ments, I have found that with certain problems there are remedies that are often useful. For instance I found that when I gave a talk to the local multiple sclerosis group, there were certain remedies that they all needed, such as Olive for the fatigue, Mustard for depression, and Wil-low for the feeling of resentment at not being able to do the things they used to. With cancer patients, Mimulus is often needed for the fear, Larch for confidence that they can get better, and White Chestnut to stop nega-tive thoughts from spoiling the quality of their life. If they are having chemotherapy or radiotherapy, Walnut is used to protect from side effects, Olive to strengthen, and Crab Apple for cleansing. We have had good results with chronic fatigue syndrome sufferers using a combination of therapies and healing to revitalize the etheric body, deep relaxation, positive visualization, and the appropriate Bach remedies: Olive for energy, Willow for frustration, and, because there is often a belief that they won't get better, Larch to renew confidence. Some patients have a good spell and are then discouraged when they feel bad again; in this case, Gentian is needed. Wild Rose is also useful for the apathetic when they feel there is nothing they can do.

Although these remedies are often needed, one must always remember that each person is a unique individual and they will need other remedies as well. I have found the Bach Remedies a wonderful tool over the many years I have used them, I am sure they are a medicine for the new age. Like Dr. Bach, I hope everyone will have them and use them for self-healing.

—*Kathleen Wingrove*

Skin Condition Case Study

A twenty-four-year-old female client initially came for reflexology for a physical condition. She said her neck and shoulders were twisted and that her skin was in very bad condition, which had been treated and controlled with antibiotics for years. She also had pains in her legs, lumps on her legs, and she worried a lot. She also had very little knowledge of the Bach remedies.

At the first session the client was so shy and withdrawn, I could hardly believe she had turned up for the appointment at all. She could not look me in the face and fiddled with her bag on her lap. She talked incessantly about nothing in particular, almost rambling. She had no confidence in herself whatsoever. This seemed to stem from the time when she was about seventeen and the onset of acne. During the consultation I used a standard case history sheet that I go through on the first visit, regardless of the treatment that is required. This covers past and present medical history, lifestyle, diet, etc. There is also a section that asks how the client sleeps and if they suffer from depression, tension, anxiety, or stress and how it affects them. At this point in the interview the client started to open up a bit more.

At the age of seventeen she was admitted to a mental hospital, which, fortunately for her, was now closed down. This was due to her constant depression, which no one could explain, other than the fact that her mother had similar tendencies. I couldn't believe the words that she used at times, it was as though she was reading them from a Bach flower remedy book. When I asked her how she slept, she said she did not sleep very well as she had mental arguments going on in her head, back and forth, making it almost impossible for her to sleep. This left her unable to get going with that "Monday morning" feeling every single day. She said that she had become less confident in herself with the onset of acne. Because of this and her constant depression she had not worked for the last couple of years, just living on state benefits.

After chatting with her a little more she rambled less, and I was able to determine that she really wanted to get better. She wanted to pursue a career in the beauty trade, even if it was just selling cosmetics.

At this point I decided to tell the client more about the remedies. She was very interested and she seemed to feel a whole lot better when she realized that she was not the only one who experienced negative thoughts and emotions. I explained that we all suffer from such feelings from time to time and that this was simply part of human nature. Sometimes we can cope and sometimes we can't so the Bach remedies are here to help us when we need it. I also explained that she might be feeling better after the first course, but that it would be wise to come back for a second interview as she might not be 100 percent cured and we might need to change the remedies used.

The remedies initially chosen were White Chestnut for the mental arguments, Hornbeam for that Monday morning feeling, Mustard for the unknown depression, that black cloud that was following her around, Wild Oat for direction, Larch for lack of confidence, and Willow as the type remedy.

I did explain to the client why I was giving her these remedies, in a positive way, as opposed to concentrating on the negative state of mind. She said just before she left, "Do you think I will feel normal one day? Wouldn't it be lovely?" I asked the client to come back in two weeks when she could have another reflexology treatment, and she could report on the results and progress of the remedies.

When she returned two weeks later I could hardly believe the change in her. She seemed much happier. She said she felt much more positive and definitely felt better due to the Bach Flower Remedies. She asked for the same remedy again. Although she did not book another reflexology treatment, I asked her to see me again in another two weeks. When the client returned there was even more difference in her. She had enrolled at the local college, and also obtained the last place available in an aromatherapy course at another college. She said that she could not believe the change in herself, she felt positive and decisive, like a new person.

I have seen the client since then but not for more remedies. She wanted me to know how she was getting on with her courses; she now attends the college almost daily. She is also thoroughly enjoying her aromatherapy course, where she has met some new friends.

— *Teresa Munro*

Difficult Child Case Study

I am not sure whether Gavin understood why he was there. His mother had just given birth to a third child and she was at the end of her rope with Gavin, seven years old. When the mother was four months pregnant the father left the family for another woman, so the whole situation has not been easy for any of them. I think it was fair to say that Gavin was awkward and hard to handle. His mother admits that he has never been an easy child.

The consultation was not carried out in my normal format. I made it less formal, but still the child was unable to answer some of the questions. With the help of his mother we were able to create a profile.

The remedies initially chosen were Holly for his anger and jealousy, Walnut for all the changes in the household—his dad leaving, the arrival of his new sister, and the fact that he was no longer the baby. White Chestnut was also added as he seemed to be having repetitive bad dreams. Larch was the type remedy.

The mother came to see me alone next time (two weeks later) to get a repeat of the remedies, since we decided not to change them. Gavin had taken three tests at school; he came first in two and second in the other. Both mother and teacher where staggered! Before this he did not have the confidence to really try, so he had failed before he started. He was also much more helpful around the house as well as at school and also generally better behaved. He also seemed to be accepting the situation with his new sister, and after several visits from his dad he was not so disruptive. Also the nightmares had stopped.

—Teresa Munro

Subtle Changes

A point that many beginners do not understand regarding the way that the Bach flowers work is illustrated by the following story.

I was running a course on the Bach Flower Remedies when one student came up to me at the end and said that she was going to purchase four of the remedies to see if they could help her with an unspecified long-standing problem. Quite by chance, I ran into her at a neighbor's Christmas party when she told me that she had taken her chosen remedies and had said to her husband at the end of the first month that she did not think they were working and that she was going to stop taking them. Her husband said, "Don't stop, I can see a difference in you." She continued for another month by which time her condition improved so much that neither of them felt the need for her to continue.

The point is that the Bach remedies are very subtle in the way that they work and others frequently notice changes before the person taking the remedies does. Another point worth mentioning is the fact that where the real source of the problem/issue is in the past, perhaps a childhood trauma, then the Bach remedies might need to work back through a long time period to do their work, and may need several months to achieve the desired result. This might especially be the case with older people.

—*Cedric Taylor*

Conflicting Personalities Case Study

Alison was a quiet person who knew her own mind. She and her husband were working through a difficult time together when she first came for treatment. She found it difficult to handle his indecision and apparent lack of direction. She was also becoming quite insecure and threatened by people on the edge of her space—children playing outside the house were getting to her and getting up in the morning to go to a job she didn't enjoy any more was becoming a real burden.

In her early thirties, Alison described herself as totally self-reliant and a loner. Yet she had always worked in a field requiring constant interaction with other people—sales. She had even become the sales office manager, and was very good at her job. She was considered "a live wire" by her colleagues.

The conversation revealed quite a conflict between these two people within her: the quiet, self-reliant person who needed her own space and became unhappy if deprived of it for any length of time; and the lively, bouncy counterpart who kept everyone else going with her energy. This was a conflict between Water Violet and Agrimony. We thought it probable that on leaving the comparative safety of childhood and school life Alison had felt, however unconsciously, that she needed to protect her inner nature from the outside world and had used the coping strategy of hiding herself behind the "live wire" exterior.

From the beginning of the treatment she took Water Violet and Agrimony, with Walnut to help protect the person who was to emerge from behind the mask. We also used other remedies to address her feelings about her husband and their situation.

After two months of treatment with the remedies, Alison was waking up refreshed and felt she had put herself back together without the hardness, that the shell had gone. Things had also changed with her husband and this, combined with her own progress, meant that she felt much more relaxed, less emotional, and at peace.

—*Judith Brooke*

Confidence Case Study

Michael and Alison were going to counseling to help them through some problems. Michael was finding it very enlightening and discovered he had a need for other people's permission to do and be what he wanted. He had also understood how much of a worrier he was, afraid of getting it wrong. In fact, his worrying had led him to ulcerative colitis and a colostomy. When he first came for treatment his coordination and balance were not good, and he found the tinnitus he suffered stressful.

A gentle person, Michael was working in the computer industry, with colleagues who were usually "hyped up" with the pressure of work. While he was good at his job, at great cost to his quiet nature, he had always been interested in the complementary therapy field, especially reflexology. He and his wife also had a dream of living in France where they had a little house, but Michael could not bring himself to make a decision on whether to break away from the norm.

For about six weeks he took Larch to boost his confidence, White Chestnut to relieve the worry, Scleranthus for the indecision as well as the problems he was having with balance and coordination, and Mimulus for his fears about doing what he wanted to do.

They went to their house in France on holiday. On his return he said the holiday hadn't "recharged him enough" and was feeling so unwell he took time off work—something unusual for him. He lost his appetite completely and felt tearful. "I've been here before," he said. We identified a lack of trust in life, a continual fear of things going wrong. We talked about how his sensitive nature found it hard to cope with the pressures of his work environment, how, in fact, his whole system was crying out to live differently. We also discussed possible future plans that would be more fulfilling for him.

In his treatment bottle this time he had Chestnut Bud to help him move forward, Centaury and Walnut to strengthen and protect his resolve, Pine to ward off any guilty feelings about doing things his way, Larch to give him the confidence to go for it, and White Chestnut to stop worrying about it.

The next day Alison came for her appointment and said, "I have a new husband." Michael had already handed in his notice and had booked a spot in a reflexology course. He was full of life, could see his path clearly ahead, he was decisive and very positively moving along it. They are now planning to take the leap and live in France in about a year's time.

—*Judith Brooke*

Abuse Victim Case Study

Sarah was a victim of abuse as a child: sexual, physical, and mental. She somehow managed to cope with this by developing multiple personalities. I have never actually met her, but her husband comes to see me. When he first came he was in great distress as she was suicidal and had on several occasions tried to kill herself, usually by cutting herself with a razor blade. She was transferred to a secure wing in another hospital. I have been prescribing the remedies for her through her husband, John.

When I first started giving them to her, we put them in a small plastic bottle, as she was not allowed glass. I gave her Crab Apple for her extreme self-disgust and self-hate and because she had no feeling of self-worth, Cherry Plum for her fear of losing control as her urges to hurt herself were overpowering, Honeysuckle to help release her from the past, and Star of Bethlehem to help her overcome her great trauma, shock, and grief.

From the outset she was pleased to receive them, as she did know a little about the remedies and in the past had used them herself. She also wrote a short note saying how she felt. I kept up these treatments and later added Sweet Chestnut to those she was already receiving as she was in such distress, and Gorse because she said that she felt hopeless.

After a month or so Sarah was taken to another hospital, which was more open. I gave her Rescue Remedy as she was feeling quite frightened and impatient to get better. Her husband told me she was feeling ungrounded and out of touch with reality and that is why I thought Clematis was needed. To this I added Crab Apple, Honeysuckle, and Walnut, the latter for the change.

The last time I saw John he said she was responding so well that she was coming home in two weeks. They both have mixed feelings about this, being excited but frightened at the same time. He felt the remedies had definitely helped Sarah.

John, Sarah's husband, also needed the remedies. I gave him Elm for his feelings of tremendous responsibility, Star of Bethlehem for the shock and trauma he was experiencing, Rock Rose for his extreme fear of what might happen, Oak because he was pushing himself to the limits of his endurance and was utterly exhausted (he works full time and also caring for three children living at home), and White Chestnut because he was unable to sleep at night.

He took these remedies for some time, later omitting White Chestnut because he was sleeping better and his mind was relaxed. I gave him Impatiens because he was feeling frustrated and irritated. At this time he was feeling much better but still wanted the other remedies as he said he still needed them.

The last time I saw John I gave him Elm, Star of Bethlehem, Rock Rose, Walnut, and Impatiens. The Walnut was because Sarah was returning home. He said he felt he didn't need Oak any more.

—*Margaret Foster*

Loss of Control Case Study

Jill had a back operation, which luckily was a great success, but she then lost her appetite and was not sleeping at night. She had panic attacks and was feeling guilty about not doing much at home; she had to take it easy and spend a lot of time resting. She felt she was losing control over her life and was impatient to get better. I gave her Cherry Plum for her feelings of lack of control, Impatiens for her frustration and impatience, Pine for her feelings of guilt, and Mimulus for her fear, which she said, was causing her sleeplessness. I gave her a repeat of these same remedies some weeks later. She made a marvelous recovery and is now back at work and singing as she takes her dog for its walk.

—*Margaret Foster*

Shock Case Study

Jane is married to a man whose brother and wife dislike her. She was going to a family gathering for a wedding, and she was terrified of meeting this brother and his wife. She was also terrified of flying. She was afraid of losing control and of having a panic attack and palpitations as she had had before. She told me she had had several shocks in her life—her father had died suddenly when she was quite young, and her mother had developed breast cancer. She said she was always anxious.

I gave her Star of Bethlehem for the past shocks, Rock Rose for her extreme fear of flying and also of meeting her in-laws, Cherry Plum because she was afraid of losing control and having panic attacks, and Mimulus because she was always anxious and nervous. I gave her two bottles to last her during her three-week holiday.

She contacted me later and said that she had felt calm during her fright and that all had gone well, and that she felt able to cope with life now.

—*Margaret Foster*

From Student to Teacher

I first came across the Bach Flower Remedies in the form of Rescue Remedy on an occasion of extreme stress in 1981. It worked when I believed nothing could possibly calm me. In 1985 friends of mine were using some of the other thirty-eight remedies to help them. Somehow I did not associate these remedies with Rescue Remedy and was very skeptical of how these little drops could be of any use to me.

In 1987 I attended my first healing workshop not realizing that this would be the start of a new lifestyle and career. The culmination of the workshop was having Bach Flower Remedies diagnosed for each of us. I went home with my bottle, took the little drops, and within four days was experiencing relief from long-standing anxiety problems. Unfortunately I cannot remember which remedies I was prescribed.

Every week I bought a few more remedies until I had the whole set and I bought some books, too. Continuing to diagnose and treat myself after about a year I began I started to suggest remedies to friends and family with a fair degree of accuracy judging by the results. For myself I found Agrimony and Impatiens as type remedies and Olive for the tiredness of being a single parent.

Over the years there have been many changes and challenges, and I have found the remedies I use most often are Impatiens, Larch, Mimulus, Walnut, and Star of Bethlehem, although at times I have used other remedies for particular issues. For example I had a domineering boyfriend and I found Centaury to be helpful.

In 1992 I started teaching about the Bach Flower Remedies with day classes and evening talks. In 1995 I gained my practitioner certificate from the Bach Centre and had a marvelous four days at the course. I am now aiming for the teacher's certificate so hopefully I can teach within the adult education system about this simple and effective system of healing.

—*B. J. Tremain*

∽

To complete this chapter, here is an interesting article by Angelina Kelly. It examines the way in which the Bach remedies help patients from a conventional medical point of view and also stresses the importance of taking responsibility for our own health. Many of Angelina's ideas and advice ring with the truth of Dr. Bach's own words. It is nice to see that "modern" healers and thinkers are supporting and advancing his theories in this way.

The Proof of the Pudding

Although, technically speaking, there is no medical or physical aspect to the Bach Flower Remedies I am aware that there are people of a scientific mind who are inclined to discredit the remedies because they cannot be scientifically "proven." These people are concerned about how and why the remedies work. Since they have not been scientifically proven there is no answer that would satisfy them, however, there is sixty years of research confirming that they do work. In an effort to make the Remedies appeal to those who are skeptics, I will attempt, as best I can, to explain the remedies scientifically.

In dealing with the Bach Flower Remedies we are working on the immune system, the endocrine system, the central nervous system and, specifically, the limbic system. The further into the nervous system we go the closer to the mind we become. The central nervous system starts in the brain and so does the endocrine system; both are very sensitive to emotions. The endocrine system regulates the hormones, affecting emotions, and when these systems are "out of order," the result is lowered immunity. When the immune system is weakened disease gets a chance to take hold. Negative, or rather protective, thinking lowers the body's immunity, therefore a strong frame of mind is essential to good health. The brain feeds on oxygen, thoughts, words, and deeds and is very sensitive to emotions; any change, even a small one, can affect the brain in some way. Therefore it is quite clear that to have a truly healthy body we must first have a healthy mind. The limbic system circles the central nervous system at the brain stem and is the seat of the emotions. It is here that the Bach Flower Remedies work directly, and it is because of this that the remedies work "scientifically."

In order to establish a strong immune system, it is very important that we feel confident and comfortable with ourselves. It is only when we love ourselves that we are able to love others, and in loving ourselves we enable others to love us too. We live in a very unsafe world where everything, including ourselves, has to be kept locked up, but it is important for us to feel safe within ourselves and within our surroundings in order for us to be healthy. The Bach Flower Remedies help us do this by overcoming our basic personality traits, to put our "problems" into perspective, and to rise above our present circumstances so that we can appreciate the learning opportunities lying within our difficulties and once again feel hopeful that all will work out for the best.

So often we seek the approval of others to validate ourselves, especially women. However, what we really need to seek is self-approval; when we have this we gradually build up confidence and self-esteem, which eventually leads to self-recognition and self-worth. When we have a strong sense of self-worth we can take on the world, confident in our own ability to cope with the situations in which we find ourselves and most of the time manage to "do what's right."

So much money and man-hours are spent on health care today. We run to gyms, saunas, aerobics, and other exercise classes, and undertake diet programs in a desperate effort to be healthy. I'm not suggesting that this is a bad thing, it gets us out and helps us to meet people of like minds, however, I suspect that it can lead to unreasonable expectations of how we are supposed to be look. I've also noticed recently an increased number of diet pills and products coming onto the market, and I really do wonder how effective they are. They are the products of an impatient, lazy society who are not prepared to work at being well. There is another way to be healthy, truly healthy, but it is not an easy way nor is it a quick way. It is, however, the most effective and long lasting way, and once mastered, takes us into old age naturally.

How do we achieve this? Well, we begin by discovering and developing peace of mind by accepting things as they are now, by forgiving ourselves, others, or circumstances for putting us here and with a clear conscience strive to make things better from here on.

We all have things and people that we value and cherish, but do we value and cherish them for the right reasons? If it is a case that we must have them, or worse control them, then perhaps we had better once again reevaluate. We must really "look" at what is valuable around us and learn to really appreciate them. Material goods and wealth are all very well but only as a means towards independence.

We have all heard the term "middle of the road" and it's not a term any of us like. Today we tend to go to extremes either one way or the other, and this is all okay for a short time;, it can be fun and even enlightening. But for overall good health it is by staying somewhere in the middle, as much as possible, that we find true happiness and well-being.

Television, movies, magazines, and books have our heads spinning with what we should be like, what we should wear, where we should shop, and how we should spend our time and with whom. We become envious of those who have more than us and sometimes begrudge them their good fortune. We look down on those who have less than we do and thank God that we are not like them. We constantly look over our shoulders at what the Jones are doing and are concerned of what the neighbors will think. We model ourselves on this star or that person and God forbid that we should ever be ourselves. But health lies in being ourselves. We must realize that to compare ourselves to others is a useless pasttime, because we are all different with different sets of circumstances, and it is this that shapes our lives and makes us who and what we are. We are all beautiful people and the sooner we realize that the better.

Listening to others is also a very hard thing to do. Countries go to war over a belief or a strip of land, families fight amongst themselves, lovers quarrel, and friends become embittered all because they are not prepared to listen to each other and appreciate that everyone has a valid point of view. We must develop and keep an open mind and listen to the views of those around us so that solutions can be reached that benefit everyone and not just the one who can shout the loudest or hit the hardest.

There are many of us who are so concerned about the future or scared of the past. It is in putting good energy and time into what is happening today, being mindful of the future, that we find success in anything we do. It is by having a good day today that we create a good tomorrow, and it is by doing our best today that we gain what we need tomorrow.

I spoke earlier about control, control of others, and I mentioned how we have to re-evaluate this. We are allowed to control but only to control ourselves. We are only responsible for ourselves, we can be responsible towards others but ultimately the only control that is healthy is control of ourselves and being responsible for ourselves. We can of course go overboard here, too, and that is not good but by being gently in control of ourselves we then exert control over our lives and this stops us blaming others for our misfortunes. Happiness cannot be bought, but it can be created and it is up to each and every one of us to create our own happiness. The wonderful thing here is that it spills over into the lives of everyone around us.

I don't know about you, but I've had a lot of difficulty believing in myself. I was never taught to believe in myself, and I certainly was not encouraged to do so. I was taught to be what others wanted me to be, nothing more was required of me. So often well-meaning parents teach their children to do as they are told and not question because they know what's best. Well meaning though this is, say it often enough and the child believes it and they grow up with no belief in themselves. This is a hard thing to overcome and for those of us who attempt it, it is usually a long and painful process. All I can say is that having done it, it was well worth the pain, and I am now discovering that I am capable of doing, for real, all those things that I once dreamed of. So again, for true health, we must believe in ourselves and come to realize that the only person we can truly depend upon is ourself. To depend upon anyone else is misspent dependence.

Religion, whatever one we subscribe to, teaches us about faith—faith in God, that is. But what about faith in life? For me it didn't teach me about faith in life and that whatever happens does so for the right reasons. It took me a long time to learn this, and I am only coming to terms with this concept now. We all know about best-laid plans, and that no matter how well we plan something sometimes it goes wrong and falls apart. This is when disappointment sets in and, if not dealt with correctly, can actually lead to ill health. Faith in life helps us to overcome disappointment, to learn from the experience, and perhaps to see how it can be done differently next time to avoid disappointment.

Perhaps most importantly we must endeavor to enjoy life. Business life seems to demand unreasonable work loads, masses of overtime, and a reluctance to take breaks. The pressures of running a home and bringing up a young family carry its own burdens and again is often the cause of unwellness. The student facing important exams often feels pressured and this can cause some very uncomfortable symptoms as well. This leads to a "from bed to work" existence with little or no time to relax and enjoy ourselves. Again, we can do this for a time, but eventually it wears us down and weakens our immune systems and this makes us susceptible to illness, not necessarily sickness, but rather, more correctly termed, "unwellness." It is important that we take breaks, that we relax within ourselves and our surroundings, and that we give ourselves time off in order to recharge our batteries.

This may all seem like a very tall order and many of you will say it's not possible. Oh, but it is! With the help of the Bach Flower Remedies we can achieve it. In a gentle, yet profound way, the Bach remedies help us lighten our mood and outlook and in this way assist us to rise above negative thoughts and emotions that drain us. They help us develop and maintain a sense of calmness and serenity, despite our tiredness and our circumstances and help us to cope with life in a more constructive way by balancing the limbic system and creating a healthy, well-balanced, functioning brain.

All of the above mentioned stress can and does play havoc with the digestive system. Many ulcers are caused by work pressure and constant worry. An acid stomach is also a symptom of churning thoughts and emotions, and anticipation/anxiety can cause "butterflies" in the tummy. Many allergies including hay fever, sinusitus, and skin complaints can all be traced back to worry, fear, anxiety, etc.

All of the above, when viewed alternatively, can be viewed as guidelines to the "science" of healthy living. Although there is no formal scientific proof that the Bach Flower Remedies work, there is research that clearly shows that many illnesses, complaints, and unwellness mysteriously "disappear" after a treatment with the remedies. Perhaps to those of you who are scientifically minded this does not satisfy your disbelief, but then I did say there is nothing physical or scientific about the Bach Flower Remedies.

—*Angelina Kelly*

Ten

Healing Meditations

The benefits of regular meditation are now well-known. We gain improved health and well-being in many ways: levels of stress are greatly reduced, and positive, peaceful, and confident states of mind are easily generated. There are many different types of meditation. Most of them relax the body and mind and promote peaceful and positive states of mind. Meditation is a simple, natural, and powerful way of realizing our abilities to become more whole, healthy, and happy human beings from within. Meditation is not difficult and it does not have to take years, months, or even weeks to master. We can even receive great benefit from our very first meditation session.

To gain the most from meditation, find a local meditation group that is led by an experienced teacher from an authentic tradition. (See appendix 1.) However, this chapter is designed to give readers an introduction to meditation and, if they follow the instructions carefully, they can gain great benefit from practicing for just ten to fifteen minutes per day.

Relaxation Meditation

This can be done either sitting or lying down and can be combined with taking appropriate Bach Flower Remedies. Relaxing music may help and you will need fifteen to twenty minutes of free time.

Begin by making a conscious intention to completely relax your body and mind, and receive whatever healing you need for your greatest good.

Take some deep breaths and settle into a comfortable position. Try to let go of anything that might be on your mind. This is your time to relax properly; it is important that nothing distracts you.

Bring your attention to your toes and try to find any tension and release it. At first it may be helpful to tense the muscles and then release them, as we need to gradually familiarize ourselves with the experience of consciously relaxing, so the process will become easier. Move your attention slowly into the rest of your feet, consciously relaxing each part. If it helps, you can think "release and relax" as you slowly bring your attention to the ankles, shins, calves, knees, etc. Continue to move your attention up through the body, consciously relaxing each part. If your attention wanders, simply return to where you were.

When you have reached the top of your head, spend a few minutes being aware of how it feels to be completely relaxed. The more you remember this experience, the easier it will become to repeat and carry forward into your daily activities.

This technique can take some time to master, so don't be disappointed if you still feel some tension after the first few sessions. This will pass in time and the technique will become natural.

At this point you can stop, dedicate your positive energy, and get up slowly, or you can continue with a simple visualization (below).

Healing Visualization

A visualization is a simple meditation using visual mental images and thoughts to induce positive feelings and a sense of inner peace. Used alongside the Bach Flower Remedies, they can greatly enhance our healing potential.

Visualize a spiraling stream of golden or white light entering through the crown of your head, filling every part of your body. Try to move the light slowly down so you get a sensation that every part of your body and every cell is filled with light energy. Imagine that your whole body and mind melts into this light, which slowly expands to fill the room, the house, town, country, planet, and, finally, the whole of space. Then spend some time enjoying this experience of pure light filling this space.

This is a good time to think of others who may need healing, people affected by local or world conflicts and disasters, or simply every living being. Visualize these people or situations surrounded by the light, and imagine that all their problems are easily transformed and healed. Then just continue to visualize them as healthy, happy, and content for a few minutes. You can think, "How wonderful, these people are now actually free from their pain and problems." Try to really believe that this has happened. Concentrate for as long as possible on the feeling of joy that arises from this thought.

Don't worry if at first this feels false or manufactured. With sincere, regular practice your motivation will become more natural and powerful. Also, don't try too hard or make your visualizations too complicated. An honest intention and a strong belief that your positive thoughts have really helped is the most important aspect. The power of the mind is limitless. By strongly imagining that through your actions people are released from their problems, this creates the causes for it to actually happen in the future.

When you have finished, visualize the light coming slowly back into the space of your body, and seal it in with a mental intention such as, "Balanced, centered, grounded, blessed, and protected." Or you can do something similar or simpler.

When you are ready, get up slowly and dedicate the positive energy you have created. Sometimes when we are setting intentions like the one above or dedicating the positive energy created through a Reiki action, it may be helpful to say or think the intention three times. This sets the intention firmly in your mind and helps you to see if the intention sounds or feel right, otherwise it may be too complicated or not clear enough. You can change an intention simply by saying or thinking a new one that applies to the same person or situation. This will automatically override the previous one, if it is for the greatest good. The power of your intentions and dedications are dependent upon the sincerity and stability of our true heart-felt wishes, so you need to keep an eye on them and check them regularly.

A Brief Bach Meditation

Once you have been taking the remedies for some time, you may become aware of the healing energy that you receive each time you take them. You may experience this as a sensation of inner peace and wholeness or as a cushion or presence of energy and love surrounding your body, a flow of energy through you, or something similar.

When you feel this happening, it is a good idea to take five to ten minutes of quiet time to sit and soak it up, and briefly meditate on the good qualities that the remedies you are taking represent. You can visualize yourself being fit, healthy, relaxed, and happy, or you can make a strong commitment to develop those states of mind that the remedies are trying to encourage. For example, if you are taking Mimulus, you can try to encourage yourself to be more confident and courageous. If you are using Impatiens, you can set a mental intention to be more relaxed and patient. If you are taking Beech, you need to be more tolerant, loving, and encouraging toward others. If you make a continuous, consistent effort to consciously develop these inner qualities, this will help the remedies work swiftly and effectively.

You can do this meditation every time you take a dose of a remedy, but once or twice a day for five to ten minutes is enough to considerably increase the healing process.

When you take the remedies, if you feel the energy concentrating in a certain area of your body or particular thoughts or emotions arise relating to some problem you have, try to relax and allow the healing energies to work for you. Just "watch" your body and mind and don't get too involved with whatever feelings, thoughts, or sensations arise; just allow them to happen and flow through you. Release in whatever way feels balanced, clear, and natural. If you can open up and trust in this way, answers to problems will simply arise, or the issue will pass more quickly than if we had tried to mentally work it out or emotionally overindulge it.

This natural releasing and healing process can happen with regard to any stressful situations that you are dealing with and also past events, even from long ago, that may not have been fully accepted or healed physically, mentally, or emotionally. With a little practice, you'll be surprised at how quickly the remedies can help you resolve problems and change you for the better.

Meditation on the Bach Remedies

This meditation is a little more advanced and can take a while to master; however, the results will more than compensate for the extra effort.

To prepare for this meditation, find a regular, daily quiet time, about fifteen to twenty minutes or more. Early morning is often best since you are fresh, and this can really help you start the day in a positive way. The room you use should be peaceful and clean, and if you have a particular religious belief, you can set up a small shrine or altar with holy pictures, scriptures, and offerings. This serves as a spiritual focal point and helps to build and hold a good quality of energy in the room and house, which is symbolic of your own body and mind. Also, if you intentionally honor, clean, and look after this space regularly and treat it with respect, you are definitely creating the karma for your meditation to gradually become clearer and deeper, with long-lasting benefits. By inviting the universal blessings or "greatest good" into your house and life by creating a small shrine, you may also notice many positive benefits in other areas of your life. Also other people may comment that your house always seems peaceful and welcoming.

You can meditate sitting in a chair with your back straight, but not tense, your feet flat on the floor, and hands resting in your lap. If you wish to sit on the floor, use a cushion and sit in a traditional meditation posture, such as the lotus position, or simply cross-legged.

Breathing Meditation

To begin, relax the body and focus the mind by mentally scanning the body for tension and releasing it. Then concentrate on your breathing, particularly the sensation at the tip of the nostrils as you feel the cool air coming in and the warm air as you breathe out. This focuses the mind and improves clarity and concentration. In fact, this simple breathing meditation, if practiced for ten to fifteen minutes daily, can greatly improve your quality of life by giving you a clear and peaceful mind. If you have no experience with meditation, it can be helpful to practice just the breathing meditation for several days or weeks before trying anything else.

Contemplation and Placement

There are two parts to meditation: contemplation and placement. Contemplation is the mental process of considering the benefits of abandoning negative thoughts and actions and of adopting positive ones. When as a result of this reasoning a strong wish arises in the mind to change your behavior for the better, then this is your object of placement; hold it, experience and feel it deeply for as long as possible.

For example, if you are taking Holly and Wild Rose for envy, jealousy, and apathy, contemplate how these thoughts and feelings have caused you many problems and unhappiness in the past. Consider how wonderful it would be to be free from these heavy, negative mindsets. Then when you feel a strong wish to release these feelings and develop the opposing positive qualities, you try to stay with and encourage these positive intentions. The key to successful meditation is to consistently make a strong inner determination to let go of negative and damaging ways of living and develop more positive, harmonious, and constructive ones.

If your mind wanders, simply return to the contemplation until that strong wish to develop your good qualities arises again, then stay with that. You are actually training and encouraging yourself to eventually think and feel this way naturally. When you "hold" an object of meditation, you should not strain the mind. It should feel natural, as if your mind has completely mixed or become one with the object of meditation, i.e., your wish to be more tolerant or patient. By regularly developing these deep wishes to change for the better, you will definitely become more positive, happy, content, and considerate. This ancient tried and tested way of dealing with life's problems, if practiced correctly and regularly, is a guaranteed solution and, unlike other modern methods of finding happiness, addiction to it produces healthy results.

The meditations will be most effective if you apply them directly to your own life based on your own life experiences. There is no point meditating every day on a vague wish to stop worrying about others (Red Chestnut) or to have less self-pity (Willow) if in your heart you are not really interested in changing or if these meditations are not directly relevant to your life. It is possible to use the technique of meditation in this way to actually suppress or avoid your most relevant personal problems, thereby actually deepening these problems—this is not, of course, meditation. You have to mentally make the meditations come alive and then carry your good intentions forward into the rest of the day. You do this by remembering the good qualities that the remedy promotes and the positive feelings and determination that arose during your meditation and try to use this motivation to guide all your actions of body and mind.

Whenever you become aware that negative feelings or thoughts, like worry or impatience, are about to arise in the mind, you can prevent them from influencing you by recalling your earlier good intentions. In this way, your wisdom and happiness will gradually increase and your daily problems will steadily decrease.

Meditation for Developing Inner Peace

You may find it helpful to try this meditation while sitting in a chair, as it is easy to fall asleep when lying down. Begin this practice by concentrating on the experience of breathing naturally, as explained in the previous meditation. This calms and stabilizes the mind.

The process of watching the mind or developing mindfulness is also a powerful way of developing inner peace and the natural intuitive wisdom that it brings. Again, a good time to practice this is when you are taking your Bach remedy. Simply look for the moments of natural peace and stay with them. When distractions arise in the mind or body, or you are disturbed by a noise, don't worry or become irritated. Simply "witness" or watch these small events and allow them to come and go, continue watching and experiencing your mind and body, and the peace will return sooner or later. Follow this inner peace and try to naturally stay with it without straining the mind, so that you become more and more familiar with it. In time, this experience will arise more easily and naturally; you will not need to consciously find or stay with it. Eventually, this natural inner peace will become your normal state of mind, and as you continue this practice, you will gain deeper and more profound levels of self-awareness and happiness.

Outdoor Healing Meditation

This is a simple and enjoyable meditation, and it is especially effective if you can practice it outside, perhaps in a garden or a park. You can do this meditation either sitting up or lying down and for as little or as long as you want. You can use a tree to rest your back against, as trees can act as a gateway, or junction, for the energy exchange. You can also combine the meditation with taking a dose of the remedies that you are using. If it's possible, sit near the place where the plant or tree from which the remedy is made grows naturally. For example, if you are taking the Oak or Beech remedy, sit under an Oak or Beech tree.

There is a natural exchange of external life force energy between a tree, the earth, and the universe, and it is this exchange that you need to become aware of and part of. In some Asian philosophies, trees are seen as symbolic or actual gateways between heaven and earth, with their roots soaking up nutrients from the earth and their leaves stretching toward the light of the sun and the energy that it gives. Indeed, Buddha attained enlightenment while seated in meditation beneath a great tree, the Bodhi tree. Trees are also seen as an example of how you should approach life. Growing steadily year by year, a tree is strong yet balanced and able to change with the seasons. It bends and does not break in high winds because its roots are deep, and it is flexible and adaptable to the forces of nature. When the conditions are right, as in the summer, its growth rate increases accordingly, and in winter it rests and recharges. Likewise, you can only be an effective spiritual being if your feet are firmly planted on the ground, and you know when it is time to challenge yourself and time to rest.

Choose a tree that you feel drawn to and place your back against it, with your feet or back between two roots if they are showing above ground. Take a few moments to get comfortable and "tune in" to your surroundings, then close your eyes and slowly relax your body and mind.

Set an intent to give and receive healing energy for yourself and others "greatest good." Once you have taken your remedy, imagine white or golden light spiraling through your crown chakra (the top of your head) and filling your body and mind until you feel completely peaceful and relaxed. Visualize this light entering the earth through your base chakra, or feet, and descending directly to the center of the planet. From there the energy radiates throughout the whole planet, touching all humans and animals, surrounding all the towns and cities, then out to the solar system, through the whole universe and all realms of existence, seen and unseen. Strongly believe that all living beings are released from their problems and blessed with this healing energy—the nature of love, compassion, and wisdom.

The main emphasis of this practice is to concentrate on the feeling of joy that arises from believing that you have directly helped others. Try to let your mind merge with an ocean of loving joy. Stay with this experience for as long as you wish before slowly bringing your attention back to where you are sitting. This universal healing is a powerful and compassionate act. When finished, as always, dedicate your good karma and, if you wish, protect your own energy system by thinking and feeling: "I am fully blessed and protected."

Mantra Meditation

A mantra is a special word or group of words that when spoken or thought have a positive effect on the mind and body. There are many mantras used in Buddhism to heal, purify, and help develop certain positive qualities of mind. The word "mantra" means "mind protection." Mantras appear as words or sound, although the Buddhist sutras, or holy scriptures, say that in reality mantras are life force energy.

One of the most well-known mantras is OM MANE PADME HUM. Roughly translated, these Sanskrit letters mean "all praise to the jewel in the lotus," although they have deep meaning on many levels. The "jewel in the lotus" refers to our Buddha nature or greatest potential for good. This arises from the lotus, which is the symbol of compassion. So the mind of compassion, or the wish to develop compassion, is the source of your greatest potential and is worth the highest praise.

This is the mantra of compassion and has a profound effect on the heart chakra.* It brings great inner peace and contentment. You can use this mantra at any time (as mentioned above) or you can receive a special empowerment from a Buddhist Geshe, or master, and combine the mantra with an especially powerful but simple form of meditation practice to develop your compassion and ripen your potential for benefiting others. For this mantra, you would need the empowerment of Buddha Avalokiteshvara, the Buddha of Compassion. Buddha Avalokiteshvara had such a great wish to help others that he blessed his own name so that when anyone one said it three times, they would receive relief from fear. This is still an effective way to prevent and relieve fear.

There are many ways you can use mantra meditations to heal yourself and others. If your intentions are truly compassionate, this is an especially powerful

---

* A chakra is simply an energy center, and the energy center of the level of the heart is especially important.

action, or karma, as the nature of mantra is so pure, holy, and blessed. You can say mantras for others whenever they need help, perhaps for people who are distressed, sick, and homeless, even for dying animals or insects, by quietly whispering mantras to them, as this will greatly help them. You can also dedicate the future effects of your actions, or karma, for their benefit. This is a special form of giving and will also increase the power of the karma that returns to you in the future.

To develop your wisdom, you would need to receive the empowerment and use the mantra of Buddha Manjushri, the Wisdom Buddha. To develop your healing abilities, you would need to receive the empowerment of Medicine Buddha (*Sange Menhla* in Tibetan), the embodiment of all the Buddha's healing qualities.

If you want to practice or know more about the different types of mantra meditations, study the appropriate texts or receive teachings from a qualified and experienced teacher (see appendix 1).

True Wisdom

One of the special qualities of authentic meditation is that it increases your wisdom. Wisdom is very different from intellectual ability. Many intelligent people are very unhappy. Since all living beings have the same basic wish to avoid problems and find happiness, wisdom is simply the ability to understand where lasting happiness comes from. As you meditate daily, you will come to see that happiness is simply a state of mind, and that since you have the opportunity to create positive states of mind through meditation, prayer, etc., these methods are the key to lasting happiness. Using the Bach remedies with wisdom can really support your progress toward this goal.

Although the essence and practice of meditation is fairly simple, it is a good idea to seek out a fully qualified and experienced teacher who can guide you along the path of meditation. If you try to learn on your own or from a book, you may encounter problems and waste time and, consequently, lose interest because you are not experiencing consistently good results. Learning and sharing your experiences with others, meditating in a group, and having the opportunity to ask questions can greatly assist your enjoyment and progress. Also, having a teacher who is a living example of what you can achieve through meditation is a constant inspiration and encouragement to your own developing practice. (If you want help in finding a meditation group in your area, see appendix 1.)

If you do a little meditation every day, good results will accumulate. You will become more relaxed and more able to enjoy life to the fullest. Gradually you shall become a true source of wisdom, compassion, and inner strength.

Conclusion

Many people believe that Dr. Bach was way ahead of his time. History shows that many great healers and spiritual teachers have been in our midst since the beginning of time. Some people might object to a comparison with Jesus, Buddha, and others like them. Edward Bach came from this timeless tradition of healers who taught that we are all more than mere physical creatures, and that we all have a great natural capacity for spiritual growth and understanding.

These great healers of humanity recognized a need in others, and they responded to that need by showing us how to solve problems and find happiness from a lasting and reliable source. Although Dr. Bach devoted his life to healing, he did not blindly confine his efforts to healing the physical aspects of illness. He discovered through personal experience, study, and intuition that the causes and cures of physical illness lie within the mind. Understanding the mind is the key to solving all our problems and fulfilling all our hopes and wishes for lasting happiness. If we depend upon this universal cure, we will find all our problems gradually diminishing, and we will naturally gain increasing inner peace and contentment from within.

Dr. Bach did two great things: he discovered the thirty-eight healing remedies, and he taught the path to inner happiness. He understood that the remedies alone were not enough to achieve the complete healing that he wished for humanity. He knew that if he was able to heal all the physical sickness in the world, this would only cure a small part of the problem. The special qualities of the remedies he discovered generate great potential for inner healing, which may lead to physical healing. However, patients have to recognize that without their own wish to acknowledge and take an active part in this inner healing, then good results are not assured.

As healers and patients, if we wish to see good results from using the Bach remedies, we must make an effort to learn more about our true nature and take responsibility for our own life. If we bury our head in the sand or fill our life with meaningless distractions, we cannot expect to find any lasting happiness or improved health. In our heart we know this truth. The bottom line is that life is short. We do not have much time, and the time we do have can easily be wasted. Dr. Bach, like all great spiritual teachers, taught that as human beings we have a special opportunity to grasp the truths of life, to understand and realize our true potential for greatness. Dr. Bach dedicated his life to healing others and spreading this message. His final message and greatest testament is written on his gravestone, "Behold, I am alive for evermore."

Dedication

To the greatest benefit of all living beings.

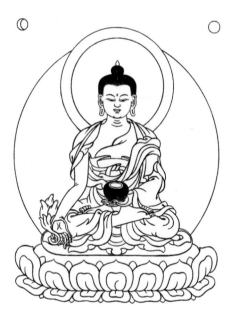

Medicine Buddha

Appendix One

Meditation Groups

The demand for a lasting solution to the problems of stress and anxiety, created by the nature of today's material society, has led to the development of meditation groups in almost every town and city. These groups vary in content and spiritual origin, so it is important to find one that you feel comfortable with, one that is run by a fully qualified teacher, and one that teaches a recognized and correct path true to the origins of meditation.

Most meditation groups can trace their origins back to Buddha, who lived over 2,000 years ago. He was born into one of the richest and most powerful royal families in India and spent the first twenty-nine years of his life living as a prince. However, despite having all the health, wealth, and good relationships he could wish for, he still felt incomplete and could see a great need in others for a real solution to life's problems. He came to understand that most people look for happiness in the wrong places. He felt sure that true, lasting happiness could be found simply by understanding and developing the mind. He decided to give up his inheritance and devote the rest of his life to attaining the ultimate state of wisdom and happiness, so that he could share this with others. All Buddha's teachings were recorded and passed down, and to this day we have a pure, unbroken lineage of the path to full enlightenment. This lineage is now firmly established in the West. We do not have to travel far to find it.

One of the largest international Buddhist organizations is the New Kadampa Tradition (NKT), established in 1976 by Tibetan meditation master, Geshe Kelsang Gyatso Rinpoche. Its purpose is "to present the mainstream of Buddhist teachings in a way that is relevant and immediately applicable to the contemporary Western way of life." Most cities and towns in the UK have a NKT local center or meditation group, and many others are opening in the United States, Europe, and all over the world. (See the "Further Reading" section for books by Geshe Kelsang Gyatso on Buddhism and Buddhist practice.) To find a Buddhist center near you, or if you would like a teacher to give an introductory talk on Buddhism in your area, contact their offices in the UK or the United States:

UK

New Kadampa Tradition
Conishead Priory
Ulverston
Cumbria, England
LA12 9QQ

Telephone/Fax: 01229 588533 (within UK)
E-mail: kadampa@dircon.co.uk
Website: www.kadampa.dircon.co.uk

United States

New Kadampa Tradition
Saraha Buddhist Centre
P.O. Box 12037
San Francisco, CA 94112

Telephone: 415-585-9161
Fax: 415-585-3161
E-mail: saraha@kadampa.org

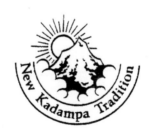

Appendix Two

The Bach Flower Centre

The Dr. Edward Bach Centre is based at Mount Vernon, England. It was the home and workplace of Dr. Bach in the last years of his life, when he completed his research into the flower remedies. Making the mother tinctures for the Bach Flower Remedies is the most important thing the trustees and helpers do at the Bach Centre. In addition, Mount Vernon has become the world center for education and information on Dr. Bach's work, including publications, special courses for practitioners, and referrals to practitioners. The Centre is open to visitors, and everything they do is to maintain the simplicity and purity of Dr. Bach's work the way he intended. To contact the Bach Centre, write to:

> The Dr. Edward Bach Centre
> Mount Vernon
> Bakers Lane
> Sotwell, Oxfordshire
> OX10 OPZ
> England
>
> *Telephone:* +44 (0)1491 834678
> *Fax:* +44 (0)1491 825022
> *E-mail:* centre@bachcentre.com
> *Website:* www.bachcentre.com

Dr. Edward Bach Foundation

The Foundation promotes proficiency in the use of Dr. Bach's system of medicine worldwide among health practitioners of all traditions. This is achieved by setting and improving standards for the competent use of the remedies, and by providing and supporting a range of educational and vocational courses and support services for registered practitioners. The Foundation gives professional status to practitioners who are working in the spirit of Dr. Bach, in the context of the Code of Practice, which provides their clients with quality assurance and peace of mind.

The Foundation promotes awareness of the work of Dr. Bach by helping members of the public learn how to use the remedies and by providing a referral service to put potential clients and registered practitioners in touch with each other. The Centre has a list of registered practitioners, and this can also be accessed on their website.

The Foundation supports the work of the Dr. Edward Bach Centre in carrying out the promises made to Dr. Bach, namely to preserve the simplicity, purity, and completeness of his work and to make it available to all the people of the world. As he said in 1936:

> *Our work is steadfastly to adhere to the simplicity and purity of this method of healing.*

Official Training Courses

The official training courses are all recognized by the Dr. Edward Bach Foundation and taught by accredited Bach trainers and, for most people, are an essential preparation for practitioner training. There are two levels to the official training.

Level One

This is an introductory seminar that provides a solid background in the Bach Flower Remedies. Even if you already have some knowledge of the remedies, it is strongly recommended that you take this course as a foundation before progressing to other levels. During this two-day course, you will take an in-depth look at Rescue Remedy and its uses, get detailed information on each of the thirty-eight Bach Flower Remedies, including case histories and practical examples, and learn how to use the remedies in everyday situations for yourself, family, and friends. You will also learn a little about working with animals and plants.

Level Two

This is an advanced workshop for participants who already have considerable experience with the Bach Flower Remedies. It gives you the opportunity to acquire practical knowledge in the use of the remedies in daily life. During the two-day course, you will acquire confidence and practice in choosing the right remedies for yourself and others, gain deeper understanding of the thirty-eight remedies and how to use them, learn about type and mood remedies, understand subtle differences between remedy pairs, and deepen your knowledge of Dr. Bach's philosophy and its application to daily life.

These two official training courses are run by the Bach International Education Program. This program has been financed by A. Nelson & Co. and developed and organized by them in association with the Dr. Edward Bach Foundation. Local offices have been set up and/or appointed by the Bach International Education Program to administer and run the courses. (**Note:** For more information on dates and venues, visit the Llewellyn website for a link to the author's website.)

Independent Training Courses

In the UK there are also courses run by registered practitioners, usually in local colleges or on private premises. They range from short half-day introductions to comprehensive courses that run over ten or more two-hour sessions. Because the Bach Centre doesn't directly control the content or presentation of these courses, they cannot guarantee that they will reach the same standard as the official courses. They are more local than the official programs, the courses run more frequently, and the cost can be substantially less, so you might find this is the most cost-effective way of taking your first steps in the use of the Bach Flower Remedies. Contact the Bach Centre for more information on these courses.

Practitioner Training Courses

The Practitioner Training Course is intended for practicing therapists (e.g., aromatherapists, reflexologists, counselors, homeopaths, medical herbalists, doctors, nurses) who wish to incorporate the Bach Flower Remedies into their work as part of their overall healing program. It is also open to people who are not practicing at the moment but intend to set up a practice in the future. It is essential that you have a good knowledge of the remedies and of Dr. Bach's approach to healing before applying. The course is constructed in two parts.

Part One

This consists of four study days, providing an opportunity to study the practical use of the remedies in depth. The program will be fairly intensive and, at the end of the four days, there will be a written assessment, consisting of an exam plus some essays and coursework to be completed at home. Successful completion of both sections will enable you to go on to second part of the course.

Part Two

This consists of a period of three months fieldwork practice in your own working environment, during which time you will be putting your theoretical knowledge into practical use. You will be required to prepare a number of in-depth case studies for presentation at the end of the three-month period together with an extended essay.

In total, the course will take about five to six months to complete. On successful and satisfactory completion of both parts of the course, you will have an opportunity to be included on the International Register of Practitioners in the Bach Flower Remedies, maintained by the Dr. Edward Bach Foundation, and be issued with a certificate indicating that you are so registered. Students will be taught the simple methods of selecting the remedies in keeping with Dr. Bach's instructions, and so those on the Foundation's register will be expected to use these simple traditional methods. Registration of practitioners will therefore take place in the context of a Code of Practice, which will set out the structure and principles of practice. Registration and certification is discretionary and conditional upon the requirements set out therein.

The practitioner course is now being taught or is due to be launched in a number of other countries around the world. Outside the UK, it is run through the Bach International Education Program, a program financed by A. Nelson & Co. and developed and organized by them in association with the Dr. Edward Bach Foundation. Local offices have been set up and/or appointed by the Bach International Education Program to administer and run the courses, which lead to the same offer of registration with the Dr. Edward Bach Foundation.

Obtaining the Remedies

Distribution around the world is handled by A. Nelson & Co. National distributors are appointed from time to time in different countries, and where there is no national distributor, the Nelson company may export direct. The main distributors should be able to tell you about local shops that sell the remedies, and about local arrangements for mail order. (**Note:** The Dr. Edward Bach Centre does not offer mail order or Internet ordering service for the remedies.)

UK Distribution

A. Nelson & Co.
Broadheath House
83 Parkside'
London, England
SW19 5LP

Telephone: 0181 780 4200
Fax: 0181 780 5871

US Distribution

Nelson Bach USA
100 Research Drive
Wilmington, MA 01887

Telephone: 978-988-3833
Fax: 508-988-0233

Dr. Edward Bach Healing Trust

The Dr. Edward Bach Healing Trust is a registered charity formed in 1989 to provide help for the relief of sickness and poverty. It makes donations to good causes and to those working in difficult circumstances to help others.

The Trust bears the same name as the original Trust formed by Nora Weeks and Victor Bullen in 1958, whose role was to hold the house and garden at Mount Vernon in trust for ever, so that the Centre would continue as the home of Dr. Bach's work. These two essential roles have been joined together in the formation of the charitable Trust so that the work of preserving Mount Vernon and helping others can continue under the same banner. Anyone who would like to apply to the Trust for assistance is invited to write to the Trustees at the Bach Centre.

Further Reading

Bach Flower Remedies

Bach, Edward. *Heal Thyself.* England:
    C. W. Daniel Co. Ltd., 1931.
Dr. Bach's philosophy of life and thoughts
on the nature of disease and health.

_____. *The Twelve Healers and
    Other Remedies.* England: C. W.
    Daniel Co. Ltd., 1933.
This book includes descriptions of the
thirty-eight remedies in the developer's
own words.

Ball, Stefan. *The Bach Remedies Work-
    book.* England: C. W. Daniel Co.
    Ltd., n.d.
This illustrated workbook combines games,
quizzes, and exercises into a complete

do-it-yourself course in using the remedies. It also introduces the basics of Dr. Bach's philosophy of healing.

_____. *Bach Flower Remedies for Men*. England: C. W. Daniel Co. Ltd., n.d.
A book which covers many aspects of the male experience: aggressiveness, love and sex, work, fatherhood, smoking, and the emotional issues associated with a range of health problems from acne to heart disease.

Ball, Stefan and Judy Howard. *Bach Flower Remedies for Animals*. England: C. W. Daniel Co. Ltd., n.d.
This illustrated book draws on insights from animal behaviorists and vets to produce the most authoritative guide to using the remedies for animals yet produced. Includes many real-life case studies.

Chancellor, Philip M. *Illustrated Handbook of the Bach Flower Remedies*. England: C. W. Daniel Co. Ltd., 1971.
A compilation of in-depth descriptions of each remedy with case histories adapted from Nora Weeks' originals, and illustrated with colored prints of the flowers.

Evans, Jane. *An Introduction to the Benefits of the Bach Flower Remedies*. England: C. W. Daniel Co. Ltd., 1974.
A useful introduction for those new to the therapy.

Howard, Judy. *Bach Flower Remedies for Women*. England: C. W. Daniel Co. Ltd., 1992.
A thorough, practical, and sympathetic book about how the remedies can help during the potentially turbulent milestones of life—menstruation, pregnancy, infertility,

dieting, screening, menopause, ageing, bereavement, sexual difficulties—by addressing the emotional aspects of these problems.

_____ . *Growing Up with Bach Flower Remedies.* England: C. W. Daniel Co. Ltd., 1994.
A comprehensive book about how the remedies can help children and adolescents—difficult behavior, sleeping, eating, going to school, family relationships, shyness, puberty, and taking exams.

_____ . *The Bach Flower Remedies Step by Step.* England: C. W. Daniel Co. Ltd., 1990.
This is an excellent all-around practical guide to the use of the remedies.

_____ . *The Story of Mount Vernon.* England: C. W. Daniel Co. Ltd., 1987.
A tribute to the work of the Bach Centre where Dr. Bach lived. Illustrated with full-color photographs.

Hyne-Jones, Tom. *The Dictionary of the Bach Flower Remedies.* England: C. W. Daniel Co. Ltd., 1976.
Shows the positive and negative aspects of each remedy.

Ramsell, John and Judy Howard (compiled by). *The Original Writings of Edward Bach.* England: C. W. Daniel Co. Ltd., 1990.
A journey through Dr. Bach's life in his own words, much of it reproduced from the original manuscripts and printed editions, with illustrations and photographs.

Ramsell, John. *Questions and Answers: The Bach Flower Remedies.* England: C. W. Daniel Co. Ltd., 1986.
Practical answers to questions about all aspects of the Bach therapy, from how to pronounce the name "Bach" to the Bach Centre's approach to conducting consultations.

Weeks, Nora. *The Medical Discoveries of Edward Bach.* England: C. W. Daniel Co. Ltd., 1940.
A biography of Dr. Bach's medical career and the story of the discovery of the remedies.

Weeks, Nora and Victor Bullen. *The Bach Flower Remedies: Illustrations and Preparations.* England: C. W. Daniel Co. Ltd., 1964.
For those interested in the botanical aspects of the plants used.

Wheeler, F. J. *Bach Flower Remedies Repertory.* England: C. W. Daniel Co. Ltd., 1952.
Suggested remedies to consider for various different moods and emotions.

Audio/Visual Items

All the following items are available directly from The Bach Centre. (See appendix 2 for contact information.)

The Original Flower Remedies of Dr. Bach. Compact disc.
Produced by an independent company in association with the Bach Centre, this is an authoritative guide to the thirty-eight remedies enhanced with some beautiful pictures of the remedy plants and sections covering the philosophy and history of the remedies.

Getting to Know the Bach Flower Remedies. 75 min.
  Audio cassette.
Side A explains the indications for each of the thirty-eight
remedies, while side B offers three different exercises for
the listener to test his or her understanding of the remedies
from the examples given.

The Light That Never Goes Out. 38 min. Videocassette.
The story of Dr. Bach's life, his career and how his work
developed, culminating in the discovery of his remedies,
with film from Mount Vernon where the remedies are still
prepared today and some unique footage of Nora Weeks
and Victor Bullen, Dr. Bach's companions and successors.
A sensitive and moving file. Available in English, French,
Spanish, Brazilian Portuguese, and German.

The Bach Flower Remedies—A Further Understanding.
  68 min. Videocassette.
Filmed at Mount Vernon, the curators John Ramsell and
Judy Howard discuss how the remedies can be utilized to
the full, explaining the differences between certain remedies and a variety of other queries that are often raised. A
most informative film that will provide an excellent insight
into the remedies for those who wish to know more. Available in English only.

Buddhism

Gyatso, Geshe Kelsang. *Buddhism: A Beginners Guide.* United Kingdom: Tharpa Publications, 2000.

_____. *Eight Steps To Happiness: The Buddhist Way of Loving Kindness.* United Kingdom: Tharpa Publications, n.d.

_____. *Introduction to Buddhism: An Explanation of the Buddhist Way of Life.* United Kingdom: Tharpa Publications, 1993.

_____. *Joyful Path of Good Fortune: The Complete Buddhist Path to Enlightenment.* United Kingdom: Tharpa Publications, 1996.

_____. *Meaningful To Behold: The Bodhisattva's Way of Life.* United Kingdom: Tharpa Publications, 1998.

_____. *The Meditation Handbook: A Practical Guide to Meditation.* United Kingdom: Tharpa Publications, 1995.

_____. *Universal Compassion: Transforming Your Life through Love and Compassion.* United Kingdom: Tharpa Publications, 1997.

Bibliography

Bach, Edward. *Heal Thyself.* England: C. W. Daniel Co. Ltd., 1931.

_____. *The Twelve Healers.* England: C. W. Daniel Co. Ltd., 1933.

Gyatso, Geshe Kelsang. *Introduction to Buddhism.* United Kingdom: Tharpa Publicatons, 1993.

Howard, Judy. *The Bach Flower Remedies, Step by Step.* England: C. W. Daniel Co. Ltd., 1990.

_____. *The Story of Mount Vernon.* England: The Bach Centre, 1986.

Howard, Judy and John Ramsell. *The Original Writings of Edward Bach*. England: C. W. Daniel Co. Ltd., 1990.

Weeks, Nora. *The Medical Discoveries of Edward Bach, Physician*. England: C. W. Daniel Co. Ltd., 1973.

Index

REACH FOR THE MOON

Llewellyn publishes hundreds of books on your favorite subjects! To get these exciting books, including the ones on the following pages, check your local bookstore or order them directly from Llewellyn.

ORDER BY PHONE

- Call toll-free within the U.S. and Canada, 1-800-THE MOON
- In Minnesota, call (651) 291-1970
- We accept VISA, MasterCard, and American Express

ORDER BY MAIL

- Send the full price of your order (MN residents add 7% sales tax) in U.S. funds, plus postage & handling to:

   Llewellyn Worldwide
   P.O. Box 64383, Dept. 0-7387-0047-9
   St. Paul, MN 55164–0383, U.S.A.

POSTAGE & HANDLING
(For the U.S., Canada, and Mexico)

- $4.00 for orders $15.00 and under
- $5.00 for orders over $15.00
- No charge for orders over $100.00

We ship UPS in the continental United States. We ship standard mail to P.O. boxes. Orders shipped to Alaska, Hawaii, The Virgin Islands, and Puerto Rico are sent first-class mail. Orders shipped to Canada and Mexico are sent surface mail.

International orders: Airmail—add freight equal to price of each book to the total price of order, plus $5.00 for each nonbook item (audio tapes, etc.).

Surface mail—Add $1.00 per item.

Allow 2 weeks for delivery on all orders.
Postage and handling rates subject to change.

DISCOUNTS

We offer a 20% discount to group leaders or agents. You must order a minimum of 5 copies of the same book to get our special quantity price.

FREE CATALOG

Get a free copy of our color catalog, *New Worlds of Mind and Spirit*. Subscribe for just $10.00 in the United States and Canada ($30.00 overseas, airmail). Many bookstores carry *New Worlds*—ask for it!

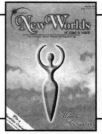

Visit our website at www.llewellyn.com for more information.

Awakening the Healer Within

HOWARD BATIE

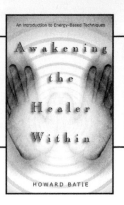

If you are looking into alternative methods of healing, you have a growing and often bewildering selection to choose from. Which healing modalities are recommended for specific ailments, and do they really work? *Awakening the Healer Within* discusses several energy-based healing techniques that have repeatedly demonstrated a positive effect on clients.

The root cause of physical disease is contained in the faulty patterns in the etheric body (the aura) or higher energy bodies (emotional, mental, and spiritual). Healing work that is performed on these energy levels can often keep disease from manifesting on the physical level.

This book discusses significant modalities for all levels of your being: physical (healing touch and reiki), etheric (spiritual surgery and reflective healing), emotional and mental (rohun and hypnotherapy), and spiritual (light energization).

1-56718-055-8
216 pp., 6 x 9 $12.95

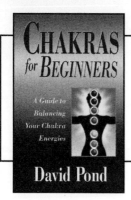

The Spirit of Healing

Venture Into the Wilderness to Rediscover the Healing Force

DAVID CUMES, M.D.

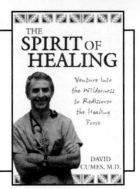

Travel to distant lands where healing is practiced in a different way: the Kalahari desert, the icy mountains of Tibet, the jungles of the Amazon, and the frozen peaks of Peru. David Cumes, M.D., leads you through primitive cultures, the natural world, ancient wisdom, and his twenty years as a Western-trained surgeon toward the ultimate discovery—that we cannot separate modern medical practice from inner healing techniques without negative impact on our health. It's an adventure that will transform your ideas about healing and wellness forever.

San hunter-gatherers of the Kalahari say that sickness resides in everyone but true illness only manifests in a few. When patients and healers both attain greater understanding of the elements of health and the "healer within," they become informed participants in their own healing journeys.

1-56718-196-1
192 pp., 6 x 9, 16 illus.   **$12.95**

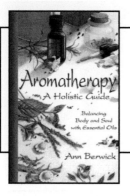

Aromatherapy

Balance the Body and Soul
with Essential Oils

ANN BERWICK

For thousands of years, aromatherapy—the therapeutic use of the essential oils of aromatic plants—has been used for the benefit of mankind. These oils are highly concentrated forms of herbal energy that represent the soul, or life force, of the plant. When the aromatic vapor is inhaled, it can influence areas of the brain inaccessible to conscious control such as emotions and hormonal responses. Application of the oils in massage can enhance the benefits of body work on the muscular, lymphatic, and nervous systems. By cutaneous application of the oils, we can influence more deeply the main body systems.

This is the first complete guide to holistic aromatherapy—what it is, how and why it works. Written from the perspective of a practicing aromatherapist, *Aromatherapy* provides insights into the magic of creating body balance through the use of individually blended oils, and it offers professional secrets of working with these potent substances on the physical, mental, emotional, and spiritual levels. ***Available in Spanish.***

0-87542-033-8
240 pp., 6 x 9, illus. $12.95

Reiki for Beginners
Mastering Natural Healing Techniques

DAVID VENNELLS

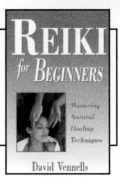

Reiki is a simple yet profound system of hands-on healing developed in Japan during the 1800s. Millions of people worldwide have already benefited from its peaceful healing intelligence that transcends cultural and religious boundaries. It can have a profound effect on health and well-being by rebalancing, cleansing, and renewing your internal energy system.

Reiki for Beginners gives you the very basic and practical principles of using Reiki as a simple healing technique, as well as its more deeply spiritual aspects as a tool for personal growth and self-awareness. Unravel your inner mysteries, heal your wounds, and discover your potential for great happiness. Follow the history of Reiki, from founder Dr. Mikao Usui's search for a universal healing technique, to the current development of a global Reiki community. Also included are many new ideas, techniques, advice, philosophies, contemplations, and meditations that you can use to deepen and enhance your practice. ***Available in Spanish.***

1-56718-767-6
264 pp., 5³⁄₁₆ x 8, illus. $12.95